Plant-Based Gluten-Free Diet Cookbook

Over 300 Quick and Simple Gluten Free Recipes for Healthy Living with 30 day meal plan included

Peter Nikki

DEDICATION
For as many who are ready to transform their plant gluten free diet experience without compromising on health

TABLE OF CONTENTS

INTRODUCTION

In Gluten-free plant-based eating is a dietary approach that excludes gluten-containing grains while emphasizing whole, plant-based foods. It combines the principles of gluten-free and plant-based diets to promote health, wellness, and environmental sustainability.

What is Gluten? Gluten is a protein found in wheat, barley, rye, and their derivatives. Individuals with celiac disease, gluten sensitivity, or wheat allergy must avoid gluten to prevent adverse health effects.

Understanding Gluten-Free Plant-Based Eating: Gluten-free eating involves eliminating gluten-containing grains and products made from them.

Plant-based eating focuses on consuming foods derived from plants, including fruits, vegetables, grains, legumes, nuts, and seeds.

It emphasizes whole, minimally processed foods and limits or excludes animal products like meat, dairy, and eggs. Plant-based diets are associated with various health benefits, including reduced risk of chronic diseases and improved environmental sustainability.

Staples of this diet include fruits, vegetables, gluten-free grains (such as rice, quinoa, and millet), legumes, nuts, and seeds. It offers a diverse array of nutrients, including fiber, vitamins, minerals, and antioxidants, supporting overall health and well-being.

Health Benefits: May alleviate symptoms for individuals with gluten-related disorders like celiac disease or gluten sensitivity

Supports digestive health due to the high fiber content of plant-based foods

Promotes heart health by reducing intake of saturated fats and cholesterol found in animal products

Helps maintain a healthy weight and may reduce the risk of obesity-related conditions.

Environmental Impact: Plant-based eating is more sustainable and environmentally friendly compared to diets high in animal products.

Requires fewer natural resources, such as water and land, to produce plant foods. In summary, gluten-free plant-based eating offers a nutritious, sustainable approach to nourishing the body while supporting your health and the health of the planet. By focusing on wholesome, plant-derived foods and eliminating gluten-containing grains, individuals can enjoy a diverse and satisfying diet that promotes well-being for both themselves and the environment.

Essential Ingredients and Kitchen Tools for plant based gluten free diet

Essential Ingredients:

Grains: Quinoa, Rice (brown, white, wild), Buckwheat, Millet
Gluten-free oats
Flours: Almond flour, Coconut flour, Chickpea flour
Proteins: Lentils Beans (black beans, kidney beans, chickpeas) Tofu Tempeh
Edamame Quinoa
Pea protein powder
Vegetables: Leafy greens (spinach, kale, arugula)
Cruciferous vegetables (broccoli, cauliflower, Brussels sprouts)
Root vegetables (sweet potatoes, carrots, beets)
Bell peppers
Fruits: Berries, Apples, Citrus fruits, Avocado
Healthy Fats: Olive oil, Avocado oil, Coconut oil
Nuts: Almonds, Walnuts, Cashews
Seeds: Chia seeds, Flaxseeds, Hemp seeds
Dairy Alternatives: Almond milk, Coconut milk, Oat milk, Soy milk
Cashew cheese
Coconut yogurt
Flavor Enhancers:
Herbs and spices (basil, oregano, thyme, cumin, paprika)
Garlic
Ginger
Tamari or gluten-free soy sauce
Nutritional yeast: Tahini, Apple cider vinegar, Lemon juice

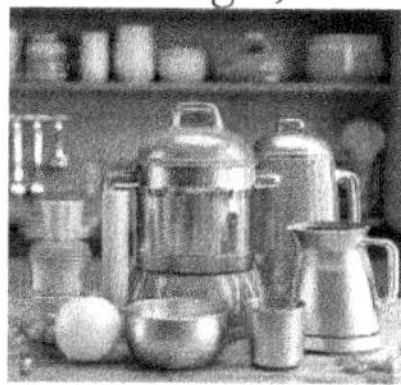

Kitchen Tools:
High-Speed Blender: For making smoothies, soups, sauces, and dressings.
Food Processor: Useful for chopping vegetables, making nut butters, and blending
ingredients for various recipes.
Non-Stick Cookware: To prevent sticking without using excessive oil.
Steamer Basket: Ideal for cooking vegetables while preserving their nutrients.
Rice Cooker: Perfect for cooking grains like rice and quinoa without needing
constant supervision.
Quality Knives and Cutting Boards: Essential for prepping fruits, vegetables, and
other ingredients.
Baking Sheets and Pans: Necessary for baking gluten-free treats like cookies, bread,
and cakes.
Mason Jars and Food Storage Containers: For storing prepared meals, leftovers,
and pantry staples like grains, nuts, and seeds.
Measuring Cups and Spoons: Accurate measurement is crucial in gluten-free
baking.

Sieve or Fine-Mesh Strainer: Useful for sifting gluten-free flours and removing lumps.
Spiralizer: Great for creating gluten-free noodles from vegetables like zucchini or sweet potatoes.
Instant Pot or Slow Cooker: Convenient for cooking grains, beans, and stews with minimal effort.

By stocking your kitchen with these essential ingredients and tools, you'll be well-equipped to prepare delicious and nutritious plant-based gluten-free meals at home.

30 DAYS MEAL PLAN

Day 1:
Breakfast: Quinoa Porridge: Cook quinoa with almond milk, cinnamon, and a dash of maple syrup. Top with fresh berries and chopped nuts.
Snack: Sliced apples with almond butter.
Lunch: Chickpea Salad Wraps: Mash chickpeas with avocado, lemon juice, salt, and pepper. Spread onto gluten-free wraps and fill with lettuce, cucumber, and tomato.
Snack: Carrot and cucumber sticks with hummus.
Dinner: Lentil Vegetable Soup: A hearty soup made with lentils, carrots, celery, onion, garlic, and vegetable broth.
Day 2:
Breakfast: Green Smoothie: Blend spinach, kale, banana, pineapple, and coconut water.
Snack: Rice cakes with mashed avocado and cherry tomatoes.
Lunch: Quinoa Salad Bowl: Quinoa mixed with black beans, corn, diced bell peppers, cherry tomatoes, avocado, and a lime-cilantro dressing.
Snack: Mixed nuts and seeds.
Dinner: Baked Sweet Potatoes: Serve baked sweet potatoes topped with black beans, salsa, avocado, and a sprinkle of nutritional yeast.
Day 3:
Breakfast: Chia Seed Pudding: Mix chia seeds with coconut milk and vanilla extract. Let it sit overnight in the fridge and top with sliced strawberries and shredded coconut.
Snack: Sliced cucumber with guacamole.
Lunch: Spinach and Strawberry Salad: Fresh spinach topped with sliced strawberries, avocado, sliced almonds, and a balsamic vinaigrette.
Snack: Gluten-free crackers with hummus.
Dinner: Stir-Fried Tofu with Vegetables: Tofu stir-fried with broccoli, bell peppers, snap peas, and gluten-free tamari sauce.
Day 4:
Breakfast: Gluten-Free Oatmeal: Cook gluten-free oats with almond milk and sliced bananas. Top with a spoonful of almond butter and a sprinkle of cinnamon.
Snack: Rice cakes with mashed avocado and sea salt.
Lunch: Mediterranean Quinoa Salad: Quinoa mixed with diced cucumber, cherry tomatoes, Kalamata olives, red onion, and a lemon-tahini dressing.

Snack: Celery sticks with almond butter and raisins.
Dinner: Vegetable Stir-Fry: Stir-fried mixed vegetables (such as mushrooms, bok choy, carrots, and snap peas) with tofu in a gluten-free soy sauce.
Day 5:

Breakfast: Smoothie Bowl: Blend frozen mixed berries, banana, spinach, and almond milk. Top with granola, coconut flakes, and a drizzle of honey.
Snack: Sliced apple with peanut butter.
Lunch: Chickpea and Avocado Salad: Mixed greens topped with chickpeas, avocado slices, cucumber, cherry tomatoes, and a lemon-tahini dressing.
Snack: Homemade trail mix with nuts, seeds, and dried fruit.
Dinner: Stuffed Bell Peppers: Bell peppers stuffed with quinoa, black beans, corn, diced tomatoes, and spices, served with a side of guacamole.
Day 6:
Breakfast: Coconut Yogurt Parfait: Layer coconut yogurt with mixed berries and gluten-free granola.
Snack: Carrot and celery sticks with hummus.
Lunch: Greek Salad: Chopped lettuce, cucumber, tomato, red onion, olives, and tofu feta cheese, tossed in a lemon-oregano dressing.
Snack: Rice cakes with mashed avocado and sliced tomato.
Dinner: Cauliflower Rice Stir-Fry: Cauliflower rice stir-fried with mixed vegetables and tofu in a gluten-free soy sauce.
Day 7:
Breakfast: Banana Almond Butter Smoothie: Blend banana, almond butter, almond milk, and a handful of spinach.
Snack: Sliced cucumber with tahini drizzle.
Lunch: Quinoa and Black Bean Salad: Quinoa mixed with black beans, corn, diced bell peppers, red onion, and a lime-cilantro dressing.
Snack: Mixed nuts and dried fruit.
Dinner: Lentil Curry: Lentils cooked in a coconut curry sauce with onions, garlic, ginger, and spices, served over brown rice.

Day 8:
Breakfast: Smoothie Bowl: Blend spinach, banana, frozen berries, almond milk, and a scoop of protein powder. Top with sliced almonds, shredded coconut, and chia seeds.
Snack: Sliced apple with almond butter.
Lunch: Quinoa Salad: Quinoa mixed with diced cucumber, cherry tomatoes, black beans, corn, avocado, and a lime-cilantro dressing.
Snack: Carrot sticks with hummus.
Dinner: Lentil Vegetable Soup: A hearty soup made with lentils, carrots, celery, onion, garlic, and vegetable broth.
Day 9:

Breakfast: Chia Seed Pudding: Mix chia seeds with coconut milk and vanilla extract. Let it sit overnight in the fridge and top with sliced strawberries and shredded coconut.

Snack: Rice cakes with mashed avocado and cherry tomatoes.
Lunch: Chickpea Salad Wraps: Mash chickpeas with avocado, lemon juice, salt, and pepper. Spread onto gluten-free wraps and fill with lettuce, cucumber, and tomato.
Snack: Mixed nuts and seeds.
Dinner: Baked Sweet Potatoes: Serve baked sweet potatoes topped with black beans, salsa, avocado, and a sprinkle of nutritional yeast.
Day 10:
Breakfast: Green Smoothie: Blend spinach, kale, banana, pineapple, and coconut water.
Snack: Sliced cucumber with guacamole.
Lunch: Spinach and Strawberry Salad: Fresh spinach topped with sliced strawberries, avocado, sliced almonds, and a balsamic vinaigrette.
Snack: Gluten-free crackers with hummus.
Dinner: Stir-Fried Tofu with Vegetables: Tofu stir-fried with broccoli, bell peppers, snap peas, and gluten-free tamari sauce.
Day 11:
Breakfast: Gluten-Free Oatmeal: Cook gluten-free oats with almond milk and sliced bananas. Top with a spoonful of almond butter and a sprinkle of cinnamon.
Snack: Rice cakes with mashed avocado and sea salt.
Lunch: Mediterranean Quinoa Salad: Quinoa mixed with diced cucumber, cherry tomatoes, Kalamata olives, red onion, and a lemon-tahini dressing.
Snack: Celery sticks with almond butter and raisins.
Dinner: Vegetable Stir-Fry: Stir-fried mixed vegetables (such as mushrooms, bok choy, carrots, and snap peas) with tofu in a gluten-free soy sauce.
Day 12:
Breakfast: Smoothie Bowl: Blend frozen mixed berries, banana, spinach, and almond milk. Top with granola, coconut flakes, and a drizzle of honey.
Snack: Sliced apple with peanut butter.
Lunch: Chickpea and Avocado Salad: Mixed greens topped with chickpeas, avocado slices, cucumber, cherry tomatoes, and a lemon-tahini dressing.
Snack: Homemade trail mix with nuts, seeds, and dried fruit.
Dinner: Stuffed Bell Peppers: Bell peppers stuffed with quinoa, black beans, corn, diced tomatoes, and spices, served with a side of guacamole.
Day13:
Breakfast: Coconut Yogurt Parfait: Layer coconut yogurt with mixed berries and gluten-free granola.
Snack: Carrot and celery sticks with hummus.
Lunch: Greek Salad: Chopped lettuce, cucumber, tomato, red onion, olives, and tofu feta cheese, tossed in a lemon-oregano dressing.
Snack: Rice cakes with mashed avocado and sliced tomato.
Dinner: Cauliflower Rice Stir-Fry: Cauliflower rice stir-fried with mixed vegetables and tofu in a gluten-free soy sauce.
Day 14:
Breakfast: Banana Almond Butter Smoothie: Blend banana, almond butter, almond milk, and a handful of spinach.
Snack: Sliced cucumber with tahini drizzle.

Lunch: Quinoa and Black Bean Salad: Quinoa mixed with black beans, corn, diced bell peppers, red onion, and a lime-cilantro dressing.
Snack: Mixed nuts and dried fruit.
Dinner: Lentil Curry: Lentils cooked in a coconut curry sauce with onions, garlic, ginger, and spices, served over brown rice.
Day 15:
Breakfast: Chia Seed Pudding: Mix chia seeds with coconut milk and a dash of vanilla extract. Let it sit overnight in the fridge and top with fresh berries and shredded coconut.
Snack: Rice cakes with mashed avocado and a sprinkle of sea salt.
Lunch: Rainbow Salad: Mixed greens topped with sliced bell peppers, shredded carrots, cucumber slices, cherry tomatoes, and chickpeas. Dress with a lemon-tahini dressing.
Snack: Sliced apple with almond butter.
Dinner: Vegetable Stir-Fry: Stir-fry a mix of broccoli, bell peppers, snap peas, carrots, and tofu in gluten-free tamari sauce.
Day 16:
Breakfast: Smoothie Bowl: Blend frozen mixed berries, banana, spinach, and almond milk. Top with granola, sliced banana, and a drizzle of honey.
Snack: Carrot sticks with hummus.
Lunch: Quinoa Salad: Quinoa mixed with black beans, corn, diced tomatoes, avocado, and cilantro-lime dressing.
Snack: Rice crackers with guacamole.
Dinner: Stuffed Bell Peppers: Bell peppers filled with a mixture of quinoa, black beans, diced tomatoes, corn, and spices, baked until tender.
Day 17:
Breakfast: Overnight Oats: Combine gluten-free oats with almond milk, chia seeds, and sliced bananas. Let it sit overnight in the fridge and top with chopped nuts and a drizzle of maple syrup.
Snack: Sliced cucumber with tahini drizzle.
Lunch: Chickpea Salad: Mixed greens topped with chickpeas, sliced cucumber, cherry tomatoes, red onion, and a lemon-tahini dressing.
Snack: Mixed nuts and dried fruit.
Dinner: Lentil Soup: A hearty soup made with lentils, carrots, celery, onion, garlic, and vegetable broth.
Day 18:
Breakfast: Green Smoothie: Blend spinach, kale, banana, pineapple, and coconut water.
Snack: Rice cakes with mashed avocado and tomato slices.
Lunch: Mediterranean Quinoa Bowl: Quinoa topped with roasted vegetables (like eggplant, zucchini, and bell peppers), olives, cherry tomatoes, and a dollop of hummus.
Snack: Celery sticks with almond butter and raisins.
Dinner: Cauliflower Rice Stir-Fry: Stir-fry cauliflower rice with mixed vegetables and tofu in gluten-free soy sauce.
Day 19:

Breakfast: Coconut Yogurt Parfait: Layer coconut yogurt with sliced strawberries and gluten-free granola.
Snack: Apple slices with peanut butter.
Lunch: Spinach and Avocado Wrap: Fill a gluten-free wrap with spinach, mashed avocado, sliced cucumber, shredded carrots, and hummus.
Snack: Homemade trail mix with almonds, pumpkin seeds, and dried cranberries.
Dinner: Quinoa Stuffed Portobello Mushrooms: Portobello mushrooms filled with quinoa, spinach, sun-dried tomatoes, and pine nuts, baked until tender.
Day 20:
Breakfast: Berry Smoothie: Blend mixed berries, banana, almond milk, and a scoop of plant-based protein powder.
Snack: Rice cakes with almond butter and sliced banana.
Lunch: Greek Salad: Chopped lettuce, cucumber, tomato, red onion, olives, and tofu feta cheese, tossed in a lemon-oregano dressing.
Snack: Carrot and celery sticks with hummus.
Dinner: Lentil Tacos: Lentil taco filling (cooked lentils with taco seasoning) served in gluten-free corn tortillas with avocado, lettuce, tomato, and salsa.
Day 21:

Breakfast: Quinoa Breakfast Bowl: Cooked quinoa topped with coconut milk, mango chunks, sliced almonds, and a sprinkle of cinnamon.
Snack: Sliced bell peppers with guacamole.
Lunch: Rainbow Rice Paper Rolls: Rice paper rolls filled with shredded carrots, cucumber, bell peppers, avocado, and rice noodles, served with peanut dipping sauce.
Snack: Mixed nuts and seeds.
Dinner: Zucchini Noodles with Pesto: Spiralized zucchini noodles tossed with homemade pesto (made with basil, pine nuts, garlic, olive oil, and nutritional yeast).

Day 22:
Breakfast: Quinoa Breakfast Bowl: Cooked quinoa with almond milk, topped with sliced bananas, blueberries, and a sprinkle of cinnamon.
Snack: Carrot sticks with hummus.
Lunch: Chickpea Salad: Mixed greens topped with chickpeas, cherry tomatoes, cucumber slices, avocado chunks, and a lemon-tahini dressing.
Snack: Rice cakes with mashed avocado and tomato slices.
Dinner: Vegetable Stir-Fry: Stir-fried tofu with broccoli, bell peppers, snap peas, and mushrooms in a gluten-free tamari sauce, served over brown rice.
Day 23:
Breakfast: Green Smoothie: Blend spinach, kale, banana, mango, and coconut water until smooth.
Snack: Apple slices with almond butter.
Lunch: Quinoa Salad with Roasted Vegetables: Quinoa mixed with roasted sweet potatoes, Brussels sprouts, red onion, and a balsamic vinaigrette.
Snack: Rice crackers with guacamole.
Dinner: Lentil Soup: A hearty soup made with lentils, carrots, celery, onion, garlic, and vegetable broth.

Day 24:
Breakfast: Chia Seed Pudding: Mix chia seeds with coconut milk and a touch of maple syrup. Let it set in the fridge overnight and top with sliced strawberries and shredded coconut.
Snack: Sliced cucumber with hummus.
Lunch: Rainbow Salad: Mixed greens topped with shredded purple cabbage, grated carrots, sliced bell peppers, cherry tomatoes, and a lemon-tahini dressing.
Snack: Rice cakes with mashed avocado and sea salt.
Dinner: Stuffed Bell Peppers: Bell peppers filled with a mixture of quinoa, black beans, corn, diced tomatoes, and spices, baked until tender.
Day 25:
Breakfast: Gluten-Free Oatmeal: Cook gluten-free oats with almond milk and top with sliced bananas, chopped walnuts, and a drizzle of maple syrup.
Snack: Sliced bell peppers with hummus.
Lunch: Mediterranean Quinoa Bowl: Quinoa topped with cucumber, cherry tomatoes, Kalamata olives, red onion, and a lemon-tahini dressing.
Snack: Mixed nuts and dried fruit.
Dinner: Cauliflower Rice Stir-Fry: Stir-fried cauliflower rice with mixed vegetables, tofu, and gluten-free tamari sauce.
Day 26:
Breakfast: Smoothie Bowl: Blend frozen mixed berries, banana, spinach, and almond milk until smooth. Top with granola, sliced almonds, and a drizzle of honey.
Snack: Carrot sticks with almond butter.
Lunch: Quinoa Avocado Salad: Quinoa mixed with diced avocado, black beans, corn, red onion, and a lime-cilantro dressing.
Snack: Rice cakes with mashed avocado and tomato slices.
Dinner: Lentil Tacos: Lentil taco filling with lettuce, tomato, avocado, and dairy-free yogurt in gluten-free corn tortillas.
Day 27:
Breakfast: Coconut Yogurt Parfait: Layer coconut yogurt with fresh berries and gluten-free granola.
Snack: Sliced apple with peanut butter.
Lunch: Greek Salad: Chopped lettuce, cucumber, tomato, red onion, Kalamata olives, and tofu feta cheese with a lemon-oregano dressing.
Snack: Celery sticks with hummus.
Dinner: Zucchini Noodles with Pesto: Spiralized zucchini noodles with homemade basil pesto and cherry tomatoes.
Day 28:
Breakfast: Banana Almond Butter Smoothie: Blend banana, almond butter, almond milk, and a handful of spinach.
Snack: Mixed nuts and seeds.
Lunch: Spinach and Strawberry Salad: Fresh spinach topped with sliced strawberries, sliced almonds, and a balsamic vinaigrette.
Snack: Sliced cucumber with tahini drizzle.

Dinner: Roasted Vegetable Quinoa Bowl: Quinoa topped with roasted vegetables (such as eggplant, zucchini, bell peppers, and red onion) and a lemon-tahini dressing.
Day 29:
Breakfast: Quinoa Breakfast Bowl: Cooked quinoa topped with almond milk, fresh berries, sliced banana, and a sprinkle of chia seeds.
Snacks: Sliced bell peppers with hummus
Lunch: Chickpea Salad: Mixed greens topped with chickpeas, diced cucumber, cherry tomatoes, avocado slices, and a lemon-tahini dressing.
Snacks: : Mixed nuts and dried fruit.
Dinner: Lentil Vegetable Soup: A hearty soup made with lentils, carrots, celery, onion, garlic, and vegetable broth.
Day 30:
Breakfast: Smoothie Bowl: Blend frozen berries, banana, spinach, almond milk, and a scoop of protein powder. Top with sliced almonds, shredded coconut, and granola.
Snacks: Rice cakes with mashed avocado and tomato slices.
Lunch: Quinoa Salad: Quinoa mixed with diced bell peppers, black beans, corn, cilantro, and a lime vinaigrette.
Snacks: Sliced apple with almond butter.
Dinner: Stuffed Bell Peppers: Bell peppers stuffed with a mixture of quinoa, black beans, corn, diced tomatoes, and spices, baked until tender.

APPETIZERS

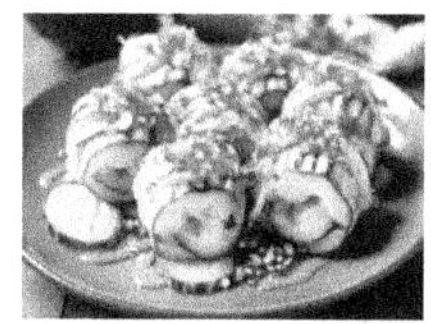

Cucumber Rolls with Spicy Peanut Sauce

Refreshing cucumber slices filled with crunchy vegetables and drizzled with a spicy peanut sauce.
Preparation Time: 15 minutes
Total Time: 15 minutes
Servings: 12 rolls
Ingredients
1 large cucumber
1 carrot, julienned
1 bell pepper, thinly sliced
1/2 cup shredded purple cabbage
2 green onions, thinly sliced
1/4 cup creamy peanut butter
2 tablespoons soy sauce or tamari
1 tablespoon rice vinegar
1 tablespoon maple syrup
1 teaspoon sriracha sauce (adjust to taste)
1 clove garlic, minced
Sesame seeds for garnish
Instructions
1. Use a mandoline or vegetable peeler to slice the cucumber lengthwise into thin strips.
2. Lay cucumber strips flat and arrange a small amount of julienned carrot, sliced bell pepper, shredded cabbage, and green onions on each strip.
3. Roll up the cucumber slices tightly and secure with a toothpick.
4. In a small bowl, whisk together peanut butter, soy sauce, rice vinegar, maple syrup, sriracha sauce, and minced garlic to make the spicy peanut sauce.
5. Drizzle the peanut sauce over the cucumber rolls.
6. Sprinkle with sesame seeds for garnish.
7. Serve chilled.
Nutritional Info: Calories: 90, Protein: 4g, Carbohydrates: 9g, Fat: 5g, Fiber: 3g

Watermelon Feta Salad Skewers

Refreshing skewers featuring watermelon cubes, dairy-free feta, and fresh mint leaves.
Preparation Time: 15 minutes
Total Time: 15 minutes

Servings: 12 skewers
Ingredients:
1/2 small seedless watermelon, cut into cubes
1/2 cup dairy-free feta cheese, cubed
Fresh mint leaves
Balsamic glaze for drizzling
Toothpicks
Instructions
1. Thread one watermelon cube, one piece of dairy-free feta, and one fresh mint leaf onto each toothpick.
2. Arrange the skewers on a serving platter.
3. Drizzle with balsamic glaze.
4. Serve chilled.
Nutritional Info: Calories: 40, Protein: 1g, Carbohydrates: 8g, Fat: 1g, Fiber: 1g

Mango Avocado Salsa

Vibrant salsa made with ripe mangoes, creamy avocado, red onion, jalapeño, and cilantro.
Preparation Time: 15 minutes
Total Time: 15 minutes
Servings: About 2 cups
Ingredients
2 ripe mangoes, diced
1 ripe avocado, diced
1/4 cup finely chopped red onion
1 jalapeño pepper, seeded and minced
1/4 cup chopped fresh cilantro
Juice of 1 lime
Salt to taste
Instructions
1. In a bowl, combine diced mangoes, diced avocado, chopped red onion, minced jalapeño pepper, chopped cilantro, and lime juice.
2. Season with salt to taste.
3. Toss gently to combine.
4. Serve immediately with tortilla chips or as a topping for grilled vegetables.
Nutritional Info: Calories: 80, Protein: 1g, Carbohydrates: 12g, Fat: 4g, Fiber: 3g

Stuffed Grape Leaves (Dolmas)

Tender grape leaves filled with a flavorful mixture of rice, herbs, and pine nuts.
Preparation Time: 30 minutes
Cooking Time: 30 minutes
Total Time: 1 hour
Servings: Makes about 20 stuffed grape leaves
Ingredients
1 jar grape leaves in brine, drained and rinsed
1 cup cooked rice
1/4 cup pine nuts, toasted

1/4 cup chopped fresh parsley
1/4 cup chopped fresh dill
1/4 cup chopped fresh mint
1/4 cup diced tomato
2 tablespoons olive oil
2 tablespoons lemon juice
Salt and pepper to taste

Instructions

1. In a bowl, mix together cooked rice, toasted pine nuts, chopped parsley, dill, mint, diced tomato, olive oil, lemon juice, salt, and pepper.
2. Place a grape leaf flat on a clean surface, shiny side down.
3. Spoon a small amount of the rice mixture onto the center of the grape leaf.
4. Fold the bottom of the leaf over the filling, then fold in the sides, and roll up tightly.
5. Repeat with the remaining grape leaves and filling.
6. Place stuffed grape leaves seam side down in a large pot.
7. Add enough water to cover the grape leaves and place a heavy plate on top to keep them submerged.
10. Bring to a boil, then reduce heat and simmer for 25-30 minutes.
11. Remove stuffed grape leaves from the pot and let cool before serving.

Nutritional Info: Calories: 70, Protein: 2g, Carbohydrates: 10g, Fat: 3g, Fiber: 1g

Broccoli Cashew Dip

Creamy broccoli dip made with cashews.
Preparation Time: 15 minutes
Cooking Time: 10 minutes
Total Time: 25 minutes
Servings: 4

Ingredients

2 cups chopped broccoli
1/2 cup soaked cashews
1 tablespoon nutritional yeast
1 clove garlic
2 tablespoons lemon juice
Salt and pepper to taste

Instructions

1. Steam broccoli until tender.
2. In a food processor, blend cooked broccoli, soaked cashews, nutritional yeast, garlic, lemon juice, salt, and pepper until smooth.
3. Serve with vegetable sticks or gluten-free crackers.

Nutritional Info: Calories: 140, Protein: 5g, Carbohydrates: 10g, Fat: 10g, Fiber: 3g

Banana Cucumber Sushi Rolls

Sushi rolls made with banana, cucumber, and rice wrapped in nori sheets.
Preparation Time: 20 minutes

Cooking Time: 20 minutes
Total Time: 40 minutes
Servings: 4
Ingredients
2 ripe bananas
1 large cucumber, julienned
2 cups cooked sushi rice
4 nori sheets
Instructions
1. Place a nori sheet on a bamboo sushi mat.
2. Spread a thin layer of sushi rice on the nori sheet.
3. Arrange banana slices and cucumber strips along one edge of the rice.
4. Roll the nori sheet tightly using the sushi mat.
5. Slice the roll into bite-sized pieces and serve with gluten-free soy sauce or tamari.
Nutritional Info: Calories: 220, Protein: 4g, Carbohydrates: 50g, Fat: 1g, Fiber: 5g

Carrot Walnut Pâté

Creamy pâté made with carrots and walnuts.
Preparation Time: 15 minutes
Cooking Time: 20 minutes
Total Time: 35 minutes
Servings: 4
Ingredients
2 cups chopped carrots
1/2 cup walnuts
1 tablespoon olive oil
1 clove garlic
1 teaspoon ground cumin
Salt and pepper to taste
Instructions
1. Steam carrots until tender.
2. In a food processor, blend cooked carrots, walnuts, olive oil, garlic, cumin, salt, and pepper until smooth.
3. Serve with gluten-free crackers or sliced vegetables.
Nutritional Info: Calories: 180, Protein: 4g, Carbohydrates: 10g, Fat: 14g, Fiber: 3g

Cucumber Cashew Gazpacho

Chilled cucumber soup with a creamy cashew base.
Preparation Time: 15 minutes
Total Time: 15 minutes
Servings: 4
Ingredients
2 large cucumbers, peeled and chopped
1 cup soaked cashews
1/4 cup fresh dill
2 tablespoons lemon juice

1 clove garlic
Salt and pepper to taste
Instructions
1. In a blender, combine cucumbers, soaked cashews, dill, lemon juice, garlic, salt, and pepper.
2. Blend until smooth, adding water as needed to reach desired consistency.
3. Chill in the refrigerator for at an hour or more before serving. Enjoy!
Nutritional Info: Calories: 160, Protein: 5g, Carbohydrates: 10g, Fat: 12g, Fiber: 3g

Caprese Skewers

Bite-sized skewers with cherry tomatoes, basil leaves, and dairy-free mozzarella balls.
Preparation Time: 15 minutes
Total Time: 15 minutes
Serving: Makes 12 skewers
Ingredients
24 cherry tomatoes
24 small fresh basil leaves
12 dairy-free mozzarella balls
Balsamic glaze for drizzling (optional)
Salt and pepper to taste
Toothpicks
Instructions
1. Thread one cherry tomato, one basil leaf, and one mozzarella ball onto each toothpick.
2. Arrange the skewers on a serving platter.
3. Drizzle with balsamic glaze if desired.
4. Season the skewers with salt and pepper to taste.
5. Serve immediately.
Nutritional Info: Calories: 30, Protein: 1g, Carbohydrates: 2g, Fat: 2g, Fiber: 1g

Sweet Potato Rounds with Guacamole

Baked sweet potato rounds topped with creamy guacamole and a sprinkle of paprika.
Preparation Time: 15 minutes
Cooking Time: 25 minutes
Total Time: 40 minutes
Servings: 12 sweet potato rounds
Ingredients
2 medium sweet potatoes, sliced into rounds
1 ripe avocado
1 tablespoon lime juice
1/4 teaspoon garlic powder
Salt and pepper to taste
Paprika for garnish
Instructions
1. Preheat oven to 400°F (200°C).
2. Line a baking sheet with parchment paper.

3. Place sweet potato rounds on the prepared baking sheet.
4. Bake for 20-25 minutes until tender and lightly browned.
5. Meanwhile, mash the avocado with lime juice, garlic powder, salt, and pepper to make guacamole.
6. Top each sweet potato round with a dollop of guacamole.
7. Sprinkle with paprika for garnish.
8. Serve warm.
Nutritional Info: Calories: 50, Protein: 1g, Carbohydrates: 7g, Fat: 2g, Fiber: 3g

Edamame Hummus

Creamy hummus made with edamame beans, garlic, and tahini.
Preparation Time: 10 minutes
Total Time: 10 minutes
Servings: 1 1/2 cups
Ingredients
1 cup shelled edamame beans, cooked
2 tablespoons tahini
2 tablespoons lemon juice
2 cloves garlic, minced
1/4 teaspoon ground cumin
Salt and pepper to taste
Water as needed
Olive oil for drizzling (optional)
Paprika for garnish (optional)
Instructions
1. In a food processor, combine edamame beans, tahini, lemon juice, minced garlic, ground cumin, salt, and pepper.
2. Blend mixture until smooth, adding water as needed to get your desired consistency.
3. Transfer the hummus to a serving bowl.
4. Drizzle with olive oil and sprinkle with paprika if desired.
5. Serve with vegetable sticks or gluten-free crackers.
Nutritional Info: Calories: 60, Protein: 3g, Carbohydrates: 4g, Fat: 3g, Fiber: 2g

Roasted Red Pepper Dip

Flavorful dip made with roasted red peppers, walnuts, and spices.
Preparation Time: 10 minutes
Cooking Time: 20 minutes
Total Time: 30 minutes
Servings: 1 1/2 cups
Ingredients
2 large red bell peppers
1/2 cup walnuts, toasted
2 cloves garlic, minced
2 tablespoons lemon juice
1 tablespoon olive oil

1/2 teaspoon smoked paprika
Salt and pepper to taste
Instructions
1. Preheat broiler. Place whole red bell peppers on a baking sheet and broil, turning occasionally, until skins are charred and blistered.
2. Transfer the roasted peppers to a bowl, cover with plastic wrap, and let steam for 10 minutes over low heat.
3. Peel off the skins, remove seeds and stems, and chop the flesh.
4. In a food processor, combine roasted red peppers, toasted walnuts, minced garlic, lemon juice, olive oil, smoked paprika, salt, and pepper.
5. Blend until smooth.
6. Transfer the dip to a serving bowl and serve with gluten-free crackers or crudité. Enjoy!
Nutritional Info: Calories: 70, Protein: 2g, Carbohydrates: 3g, Fat: 6g, Fiber: 1g

Cauliflower Buffalo Wings

Crispy cauliflower florets tossed in spicy buffalo sauce, perfect for game day or any gathering.
Preparation Time: 15 minutes
Cooking Time: 25 minutes
Total Time: 40 minutes
Servings: 4
Ingredients
1 head cauliflower, cut into florets
1/2 cup gluten-free all-purpose flour
1/2 cup water
1 teaspoon garlic powder
1/2 teaspoon paprika
Salt and pepper to taste
1/2 cup hot sauce
2 tablespoons vegan butter, melted
Celery sticks and dairy-free ranch dressing for serving
Instructions
1. Preheat oven to 450°F (230°C).
2. Line a baking sheet with parchment paper.
3. In a large bowl, whisk together gluten-free flour, water, garlic powder, paprika, salt, and pepper to make a batter.
4. Dip cauliflower florets into the batter, shaking off excess, and place them on the prepared baking sheet.
5. Bake for 20 minutes, flipping halfway through, until cauliflower is golden and crispy.
6. In a separate bowl, combine hot sauce and melted vegan butter to make buffalo sauce.
7. Toss the baked cauliflower in buffalo sauce until well coated.
8. Return cauliflower to the baking sheet and bake for an additional 5 minutes.
9. Serve hot with celery sticks and dairy-free ranch dressing.
Nutritional Info: Calories: 120, Protein: 3g, Carbohydrates: 14g, Fat: 6g, Fiber: 3g

Sushi Rolls

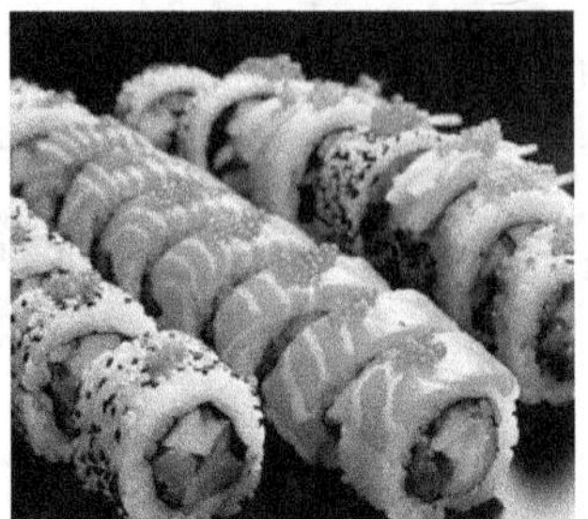

Homemade sushi rolls filled with avocado, cucumber, carrot, and tofu, perfect for a sushi night at home.

Preparation Time: 30 minutes

Total Time: 30 minutes

Servings: 4 rolls

Ingredients

4 nori seaweed sheets

2 cups cooked sushi rice

1 avocado, sliced

1/2 cucumber, julienned

1 carrot, julienned

4 oz firm tofu, sliced into thin strips

Wasabi, soy sauce, and pickled ginger for serving

Instructions

1. Place a nori sheet shiny side down on a bamboo sushi mat.

2. Spread a thin layer of sushi rice evenly over the nori sheet, leaving about 1 inch of space at the top.

3. Arrange avocado slices, cucumber, carrot, and tofu strips horizontally across the bottom third of the rice.

4. Lift the bottom edge of the sushi mat and roll it tightly over the filling, using your fingers to tuck and tighten the roll.

5. Continue rolling until you reach the top edge of the nori sheet.

6. Moisten the top edge of the nori sheet with water to seal the roll.

7. Repeat with the remaining nori sheets and filling ingredients.

8. Use a sharp knife to slice each roll into bite-sized pieces.

9. Serve with soy sauce, wasabi, and pickled ginger.

Nutritional Info: Calories: 220, Protein: 6g, Carbohydrates: 38g, Fat: 5g, Fiber: 5g

Crispy Tofu Bites

Bite-sized tofu cubes coated in a crispy gluten-free breading, perfect for dipping.

Preparation Time: 15 minutes

Cooking Time: 20 minutes
Total Time: 35 minutes
Servings: 4
Ingredients
1 block firm tofu (14 oz.) pressed and cubed
1/2 cup gluten-free breadcrumbs
1/4 cup cornmeal
1 teaspoon garlic powder
1 teaspoon smoked paprika
1/2 teaspoon onion powder
Salt and pepper to taste
2 tablespoons olive oil
Instructions
1. Preheat oven to 400°F (200°C).
2. Line a baking sheet with parchment paper.
3. In a shallow dish, combine gluten-free breadcrumbs, cornmeal, garlic powder, smoked paprika, onion powder, salt, and pepper.
4. Toss tofu cubes in olive oil until evenly coated.
5. Dip each tofu cube into the breadcrumb mixture, pressing gently to adhere.
6. Place coated tofu cubes on the prepared baking sheet.
7. Bake for 20-25 minutes until golden and crispy, flipping halfway through.
8. Serve hot with your favorite dipping sauce.
Nutritional Info: Calories: 180, Protein: 10g, Carbohydrates: 15g, Fat: 8g, Fiber: 3g

Roasted Vegetable Bruschetta

Toasted gluten-free baguette slices topped with roasted vegetables and balsamic glaze.
Preparation Time: 15 minutes
Cooking Time: 25 minutes
Total Time: 40 minutes
Servings: About 12 bruschetta
Ingredients
1 gluten-free baguette, sliced
1 cup cherry tomatoes, halved
1 small zucchini, diced
1 small yellow squash, diced
1 red bell pepper, diced
1 tablespoon olive oil
Salt and pepper to taste
Balsamic glaze for drizzling
Fresh basil leaves for garnish
Instructions
1. Preheat oven to 400°F (200°C).
2. Line a baking sheet with parchment paper.
3. Arrange sliced baguette on the prepared baking sheet.
4. In a bowl, toss cherry tomatoes, diced zucchini, yellow squash, and red bell pepper with olive oil, salt, and pepper.

5. Spread the vegetables in a single layer on another baking sheet.
6. Roast both the baguette slices and the vegetables in the preheated oven for 20-25 minutes until bread is toasted and vegetables are tender.
7. Top each baguette slice with roasted vegetables.
8. Garnish with fresh basil leaves and drizzle with balsamic glaze. Serve and enjoy immediately
Nutritional Info: Calories: 70, Protein: 2g, Carbohydrates: 12g, Fat: 2g, Fiber: 2g

Broccoli Cashew Stir-Fry

Stir-fried broccoli and cashews in a savory sauce.
Preparation Time: 10 minutes
Cooking Time: 15 minutes
Total Time: 25 minutes
Servings: 4
Ingredients
2 cups broccoli florets
1/2 cup soaked cashews
2 tablespoons soy sauce or tamari
1 tablespoon maple syrup
1 tablespoon sesame oil
2 cloves garlic, minced
1 teaspoon grated ginger
Cooked rice or quinoa for serving
Instructions
1. Heat the oil in a large skillet over medium-high heat.
2. Add minced garlic and grated ginger, and sauté until fragrant.
3. Add broccoli florets and soaked cashews to the skillet, and stir-fry for 5-7 minutes, or until broccoli is tender-crisp.
4. In a small bowl, whisk together soy sauce and maple syrup, then pour over the broccoli and cashews.
5. Cook for an additional 2-3 minutes, until the sauce has thickened.
6. Serve over cooked rice or quinoa.
Nutritional Info: Calories: 250, Protein: 8g, Carbohydrates: 20g, Fat: 14g, Fiber: 4g

Stuffed Mushroom Caps

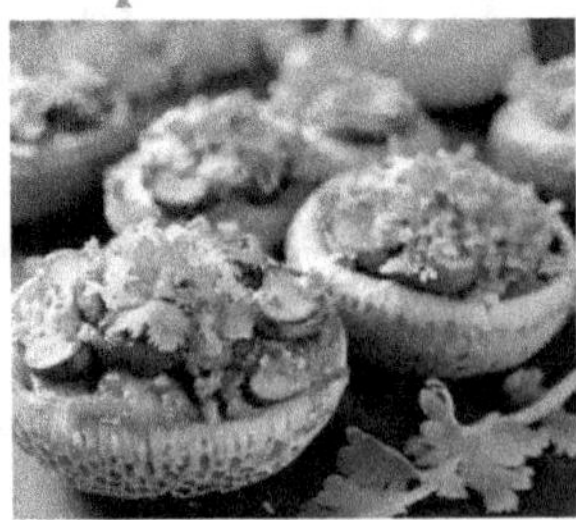

Juicy mushroom caps stuffed with a flavorful mixture of quinoa, spinach, and spices.
Preparation Time: 15 minutes

Cooking Time: 20 minutes
Total Time: 35 minutes
Servings: 12
Ingredients
12 large mushroom caps
1/2 cup cooked quinoa
1 cup chopped spinach
1/4 cup diced onion
2 cloves garlic, minced
1/4 teaspoon dried thyme
Salt and pepper to taste
Olive oil for brushing
Instructions
1. Preheat oven to 375°F (190°C).
2. Line a baking sheet with parchment paper.
3. Remove stems from mushroom caps and place caps on the prepared baking sheet.
4. In a skillet, sauté onion and garlic until softened. Add the spinach and cook until wilted.
5. Stir in cooked quinoa, dried thyme, salt, and pepper. Cook for another 2 minutes.
6. Spoon the quinoa mixture into each mushroom cap, pressing gently to pack.
7. Brush the tops of stuffed mushrooms with olive oil.
8. Bake for 18-20 minutes until mushrooms are tender.
9. Serve hot.
Nutritional Info: Calories: 80, Protein: 4g, Carbohydrates: 12g, Fat: 2g, Fiber: 3g

Zucchini Fritters

Crispy fritters made with grated zucchini, chickpea flour, and aromatic spices.
Preparation Time: 20 minutes
Cooking Time: 15 minutes
Total Time: 35 minutes
Servings: 12 fritters
Ingredients
2 medium zucchinis, grated
1/2 cup chickpea flour
2 tablespoons nutritional yeast
2 cloves garlic, minced
1 teaspoon ground cumin
1/2 teaspoon smoked paprika
Salt and pepper to taste
Olive oil for frying
Instructions
1. Place grated zucchini in a clean kitchen towel and squeeze out excess moisture.

2. In a large bowl, combine grated zucchini, chickpea flour, nutritional yeast, minced garlic, ground cumin, smoked paprika, salt, and pepper. Mix well to form a batter.
3. Heat olive oil in a skillet over medium heat.
4. Drop spoonful of the batter into the skillet and use back of a spoon to slightly it.
5. Cook for 3-4 minutes on each side until golden brown and crispy.
6. Transfer cooked fritters to a paper towel-lined plate to drain excess oil.
7. Serve the fritters hot with your favorite dipping sauce.
Nutritional Info: Calories: 60, Protein: 3g, Carbohydrates: 8g, Fat: 2g, Fiber: 2g

Spinach Artichoke Dip

Creamy dip loaded with spinach, artichoke hearts, and dairy-free cheese, perfect for sharing.
Preparation Time: 15 minutes
Cooking Time: 25 minutes
Total Time: 40 minutes
Servings: About 2 cups

Ingredients
1 cup cooked spinach, chopped
1 can artichoke hearts (14 oz.) drained and chopped
1/2 cup dairy-free cream cheese
1/2 cup dairy-free mayonnaise
1/4 cup nutritional yeast
2 cloves garlic, minced
Salt and pepper to taste
Gluten-free tortilla chips or crudité for serving

Instructions
1. Preheat oven to 375°F (190°C). Grease a baking dish.
2. In a mixing bowl, combine chopped spinach, chopped artichoke hearts, dairy-free cream cheese, dairy-free mayonnaise, nutritional yeast, minced garlic, salt, and pepper.
3. Transfer the mixture to the prepared baking dish and spread it out evenly.
4. Bake for 20-25 minutes until bubbly and golden brown on top.
5. Serve hot with gluten-free tortilla chips or crudité.
Nutritional Info: Calories: 120, Protein: 3g, Carbohydrates: 6g, Fat: 10g, Fiber: 3g

Broccoli Bites

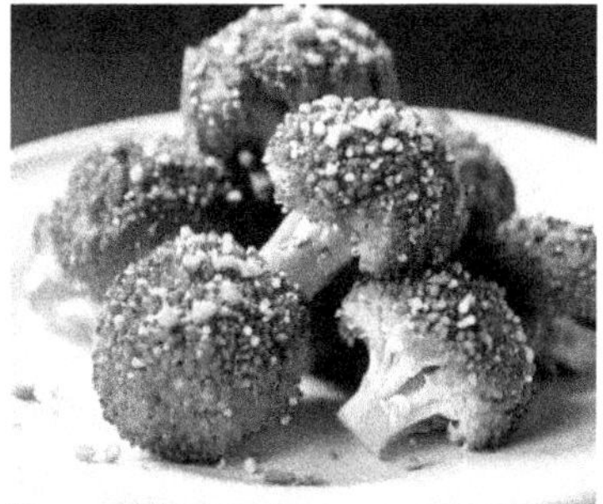

Crispy broccoli florets coated in gluten-free breadcrumbs.
Preparation Time: 15 minutes
Cooking Time: 20 minutes
Total Time: 35 minutes
Servings: 4
Ingredients
2 cups broccoli florets
1/2 cup gluten-free breadcrumbs
2 tablespoons nutritional yeast
1/2 teaspoon garlic powder
Salt and pepper to taste
Instructions
1. Preheat oven to 375°F (190°C).
2. In a bowl, mix breadcrumbs, nutritional yeast, garlic powder, salt, and pepper.
3. Dip broccoli florets in the breadcrumb mixture, ensuring they're coated evenly.
4. Place coated broccoli on a baking sheet and bake for 20 minutes or until crispy.
Nutritional Info: Calories: 120, Protein: 6g, Carbohydrates: 20g, Fat: 2g, Fiber: 5g

Banana Walnut Bites

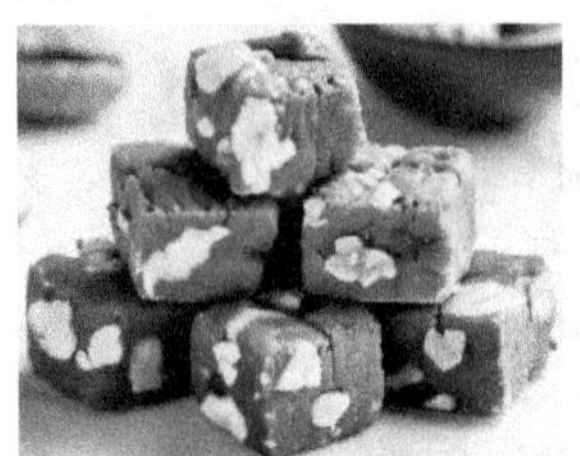

Sliced bananas topped with creamy cashew butter and crushed walnuts.
Preparation Time: 10 minutes
Servings: 4
Ingredients
2 bananas, sliced
1/4 cup cashew butter
1/4 cup crushed walnuts
Instructions
1. Spread cashew butter on banana slices.
2. Sprinkle crushed walnuts on top.
3. Serve immediately.
Nutritional Info: Calories: 180, Protein: 4g, Carbohydrates: 20g, Fat: 10g, Fiber: 3g

Cucumber Cashew Rolls

Thinly sliced cucumber filled with creamy cashew cheese.
Preparation Time: 15 minutes
Servings: 4
Ingredients
1 large cucumber
1 cup soaked cashews
2 tablespoons lemon juice
1 clove garlic
Salt and pepper to taste
Instructions
1. Blend soaked cashews, lemon juice, garlic, salt, and pepper until smooth.
2. Use a mandoline or vegetable peeler to slice the cucumber lengthwise.
3. Spread cashew cheese on cucumber slices and roll them up.
4. Secure with toothpicks if needed.
Nutritional Info: Calories: 150, Protein: 5g, Carbohydrates: 10g, Fat: 8g, Fiber: 2g

Carrot Cashew Hummus

Creamy hummus made with carrots and cashews.
Preparation Time: 10 minutes
Cooking Time: 20 minutes
Total Time: 30 minutes
Servings: 4
Ingredients

2 cups chopped carrots
1/2 cup soaked cashews
2 tablespoons tahini
2 tablespoons lemon juice
1 clove garlic
2 tablespoons olive oil
Salt and pepper to taste
Instructions
1. Steam carrots until tender.
2. In a food processor, blend cooked carrots, soaked cashews, tahini, lemon juice, garlic, olive oil, salt, and pepper until smooth.
3. Serve with sliced vegetables or gluten-free crackers.
Nutritional Info: Calories: 180, Protein: 5g, Carbohydrates: 10g, Fat: 14g, Fiber: 3g

Walnut-Stuffed Dates

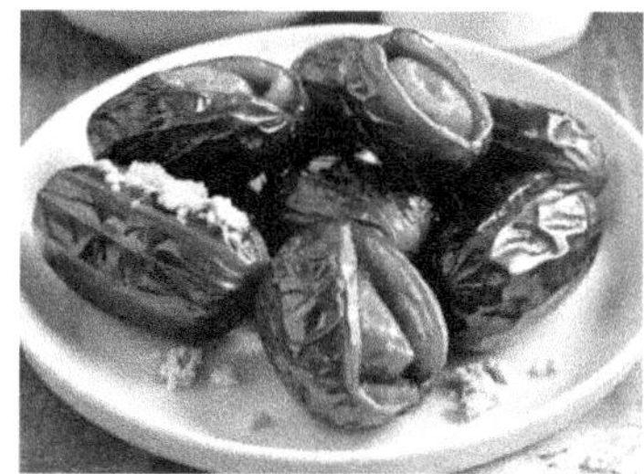

Medjool dates stuffed with walnuts.
Preparation Time: 5 minutes
Servings: 4
Ingredients
8 Medjool dates
16 walnut halves
Instructions
1. Make a lengthwise incision in each date and remove the pit.
2. Stuff each date with two walnut halves.
3. Serve immediately.
Nutritional Info: Calories: 160, Protein: 2g, Carbohydrates: 40g, Fat: 4g, Fiber: 5g

Smoothie Bowl

Creamy smoothie bowl made with banana and cashews, topped with sliced fruit and nuts.
Preparation Time: 10 minutes
Total Time: 10 minutes
Servings: 2
Ingredients
2 ripe bananas, frozen
1/2 cup soaked cashews
1/2 cup almond milk
Toppings: sliced banana, chopped walnuts, shredded coconut

Instructions
1. In a blender, combine frozen bananas, soaked cashews, and almond milk.
2. Blend until smooth and creamy.
3. Pour into bowls and top with sliced banana, chopped walnuts, and shredded coconut.
4. Serve immediately.
Nutritional Info: Calories: 280, Protein: 7g, Carbohydrates: 40g, Fat: 12g, Fiber: 6g

Walnut Banana Pancakes

Fluffy pancakes made with ripe bananas and crushed walnuts.
Preparation Time: 10 minutes
Cooking Time: 15 minutes
Total Time: 25 minutes
Serving: 4
Ingredients
2 ripe bananas, mashed
1 cup gluten-free pancake mix
1/2 cup chopped walnuts
1 cup almond milk
1 tablespoon maple syrup
1 teaspoon vanilla extract
Coconut oil for cooking
Instructions
1. In a bowl, mix mashed bananas, pancake mix, chopped walnuts, almond milk, maple syrup, and vanilla extract until well combined.
2. Heat a skillet over medium heat and lightly grease with coconut oil.
3. Pour 1/4 cup of batter onto the skillet for each pancake.
4. Cook until bubbles form on the surface, then flip and cook until golden brown.
5. Serve warm with maple syrup and sliced bananas.
Nutritional Info: Calories: 280, Protein: 6g, Carbohydrates: 40g, Fat: 10g, Fiber: 5g

BREAKFAST

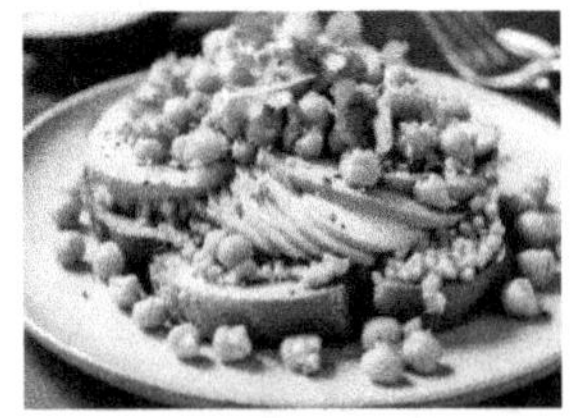

Avocado Toast with Chickpea Scramble

Creamy avocado paired with protein-packed chickpea scramble on gluten-free toast.
Preparation Time: 10 minutes

Cooking Time: 10 minutes
Total Time: 20 minutes
Servings: 2
Ingredients
4 slices gluten-free bread
1 ripe avocado
1 can (15 oz) chickpeas, drained and rinsed
1 tablespoon olive oil
1/2 teaspoon ground cumin
1/2 teaspoon turmeric
Salt and pepper to taste
Optional toppings: cherry tomatoes, fresh herbs
Instructions
1. Mash the avocado in a bowl and season with salt and pepper.
2. In a skillet, heat olive oil over medium heat. Add chickpeas, cumin, turmeric, salt, and pepper.
3. Cook for 5-7 minutes until chickpeas are slightly crispy.
4. Toast the gluten-free bread slices.
5. Spread mashed avocado on each toast and top with chickpea scramble.
6. Garnish with cherry tomatoes and fresh herbs if desired.
Nutritional Info: Calories: 280, Protein: 10g, Carbohydrates: 30g, Fat: 15g, Fiber: 10g

Chia Seed Pudding with Mixed Berries

A creamy and nutritious pudding made with chia seeds and served with a medley of fresh berries.
Preparation Time: 5 minutes
Cooking Time: 0 minutes
Total Time: 5 minutes (+overnight chilling)
Servings: 2
Ingredients
1/4 cup chia seeds
1 cup unsweetened almond milk
1 tablespoon maple syrup or agave nectar
1/2 teaspoon vanilla extract
1 cup mixed berries (such as strawberries, blueberries, raspberries)
Optional toppings: sliced almonds, coconut flakes
Instructions
1. In a bowl, whisk together chia seeds, almond milk, maple syrup, and vanilla extract.
2. Let it sit for 5 minutes, then whisk again to prevent clumping.
3. Cover the bowl and refrigerate overnight or for at least 4 hours until the mixture thickens and becomes pudding-like.
4. Stir the chia pudding before serving and divide it into bowls.
5. Top with mixed berries and optional toppings.
Nutritional Info: Calories: 220, Protein: 6g, Carbohydrates: 25g, Fat: 10g, Fiber: 12g

Smoothie Bowl with Spinach, Banana, and Almond Butter

A vibrant and nutrient-packed bowl featuring a smoothie base of spinach and banana, topped with almond butter and seeds.

Preparation Time: 10 minutes
Cooking Time: 0 minutes
Total Time: 10 minutes
Servings: 2

Ingredients

2 cups fresh spinach
2 ripe bananas, sliced and frozen
1/4 cup almond milk
2 tablespoons almond butter
1 tablespoon chia seeds
1 tablespoon hemp seeds
Fresh fruit for topping (such as sliced banana, berries)

Instructions

1. In a blender, combine fresh spinach, frozen banana slices, and almond milk. Blend until smooth and creamy.
2. Pour the smoothie into bowls.
3. Drizzle almond butter on top and sprinkle with chia seeds and hemp seeds.
4. Add fresh fruit as desired.

Nutritional Info: Calories: 300, Protein: 8g, Carbohydrates: 40g, Fat: 15g, Fiber: 10g

Quinoa Breakfast Bowl with Coconut Milk and Mango

A hearty and tropical breakfast bowl featuring cooked quinoa, creamy coconut milk, and sweet mango.

Preparation Time: 5 minutes
Cooking Time: 15 minutes
Total Time: 20 minutes
Servings: 2

Ingredients

1 cup cooked quinoa
1 cup coconut milk
1 ripe mango, diced
2 tablespoons shredded coconut
2 tablespoons chopped nuts (such as almonds or cashews)
Optional sweetener: maple syrup or agave nectar

Instructions

1. In a small saucepan, heat coconut milk until warm.
2. Divide cooked quinoa into bowls.
3. Pour warm coconut milk over the quinoa.
4. Top with diced mango, shredded coconut, and chopped nuts.
5. Sweeten with maple syrup or agave nectar if desired.

Nutritional Info: Calories: 320, Protein: 6g, Carbohydrates: 45g, Fat: 12g, Fiber: 7g

Banana Buckwheat Pancakes with Blueberry Compote

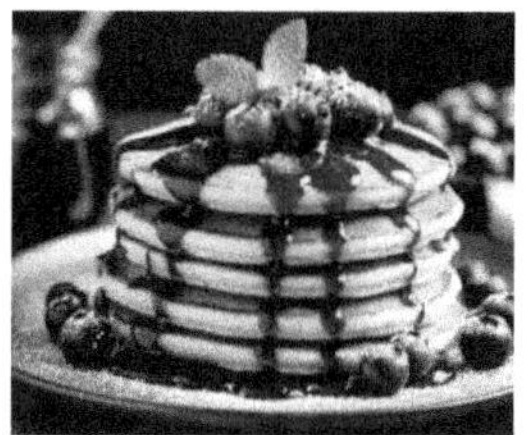

Fluffy gluten-free pancakes made with buckwheat flour and served with a warm blueberry compote.
Preparation Time: 10 minutes
Cooking Time: 15 minutes
Total Time: 25 minutes
Servings: 2
Ingredients
1 cup buckwheat flour
1 ripe banana, mashed
1 tablespoon maple syrup
1 teaspoon baking powder
1/2 teaspoon cinnamon
Pinch of salt
1/2 cup unsweetened almond milk
Coconut oil for cooking
For the blueberry compote:
1 cup fresh or frozen blueberries
1 tablespoon maple syrup
Juice of 1/2 lemon
Instructions
1. In a bowl, mix together buckwheat flour, mashed banana, maple syrup, baking powder, cinnamon, salt, and almond milk until smooth.
2. Heat coconut oil in a non-stick skillet over medium heat.
3. Pour 1/4 cup of batter onto the skillet for each pancake.
4. Cook for 2-3 minutes on each side, or until golden brown.
5. For the blueberry compote, combine blueberries, maple syrup, and lemon juice in a small saucepan. Cook over medium heat until berries burst and the mixture thickens.
6. Serve pancakes with warm blueberry compote.
Nutritional Info: Calories: 300, Protein: 6g, Carbohydrates: 45g, Fat: 10g, Fiber: 8g
Coconut Yogurt Parfait with Granola and Mixed Berries
A refreshing parfait made with dairy-free coconut yogurt, crunchy granola, and fresh berries.
Preparation Time: 5 minutes
Cooking Time: 0 minutes
Total Time: 5 minutes
Serving: 1
Ingredients

1/2 cup dairy-free coconut yogurt
1/4 cup gluten-free granola
1/2 cup mixed berries (such as strawberries, blueberries, raspberries)
Optional toppings: shredded coconut, sliced almonds
Instructions
1. In a glass or bowl, layer coconut yogurt, granola, and mixed berries.
2. Repeat layers until ingredients are used up.
3. Top with shredded coconut and sliced almonds if desired.
Nutritional Info: Calories: 280, Protein: 5g, Carbohydrates: 40g, Fat: 10g, Fiber: 8g

Tofu Scramble Breakfast Tacos

Flavorful tofu scramble wrapped in gluten-free tortillas and topped with avocado and salsa.
Preparation Time: 10 minutes
Cooking Time: 10 minutes
Total Time: 20 minutes
Servings: 2
Ingredients
1 block firm tofu, drained and crumbled
1 tablespoon olive oil
1/2 onion, diced
1 bell pepper, diced
1 teaspoon ground cumin
1/2 teaspoon turmeric
Salt and pepper to taste
4 gluten-free tortillas
1 ripe avocado, sliced
Salsa for serving
Instructions
1. Heat olive oil in a skillet over medium-high heat.
2. Add diced onion and bell pepper, sauté until softened.
3. Add crumbled tofu to the skillet, along with ground cumin, turmeric, salt, and pepper.
4. Cook for 5-7 minutes until tofu is heated through and well combined with the spices.
5. Warm gluten-free tortillas in a dry skillet or microwave.
6. Divide tofu scramble among the tortillas.
7. Top with sliced avocado and salsa.
Nutritional Info: Calories: 320, Protein: 12g, Carbohydrates: 35g, Fat: 15g, Fiber: 10g

Green Smoothie with Kale, Pineapple, and Ginger

A refreshing green smoothie packed with kale, tropical pineapple, and zesty ginger.
Preparation Time: 5 minutes
Cooking Time: 0 minutes
Total Time: 5 minutes
Servings: 1
Ingredients

1 cup chopped kale leaves, stems removed
1 cup frozen pineapple chunks
1/2 inch piece of fresh ginger, peeled
1 ripe banana
1 cup unsweetened coconut water or almond milk
Optional: 1 tablespoon chia seeds or flaxseeds
Instructions
1. Place kale, frozen pineapple chunks, fresh ginger, banana, and coconut water or almond milk in a blender.
2. Blend until smooth and creamy.
3. If desired, add chia seeds or flaxseeds and blend again briefly.
4. Pour into a glass and serve immediately.
Nutritional Info: Calories: 250, Protein: 5g, Carbohydrates: 40g, Fat: 8g, Fiber: 6g

Sweet Potato and Black Bean Breakfast Hash

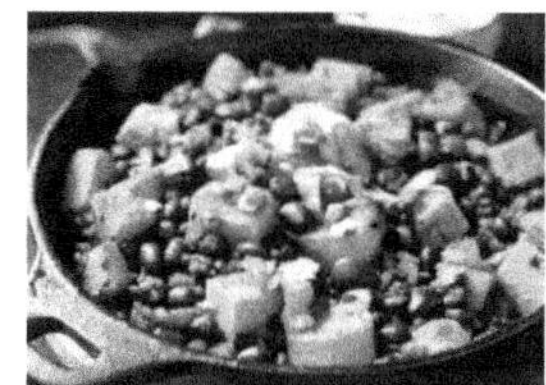

A hearty breakfast hash made with sweet potatoes, black beans, and flavorful spices.
Preparation Time: 10 minutes
Cooking Time: 20 minutes
Total Time: 30 minutes
Servings: 2
Ingredients
2 medium sweet potatoes, peeled and diced
1 can (15 oz) black beans, drained and rinsed
1/2 onion, diced
1 bell pepper, diced
2 cloves garlic, minced
1 teaspoon ground cumin
1/2 teaspoon smoked paprika
Salt and pepper to taste
2 tablespoons olive oil
Fresh cilantro for garnish
Instructions
1. Heat olive oil in a skillet over medium heat.
2. Add diced sweet potatoes and cook until softened and slightly browned, about 10 minutes.
3. Add diced onion, bell pepper, and minced garlic to the skillet. Cook until vegetables are tender.
4. Stir in black beans, ground cumin, smoked paprika, salt, and pepper.
5. Cook for another 5 minutes to heat through and allow flavors to meld.
6. Serve hot, garnished with fresh cilantro.

Nutritional Info: Calories: 300, Protein: 8g, Carbohydrates: 45g, Fat: 10g, Fiber: 10g

Vegan Banana Bread

Moist and delicious banana bread made with gluten-free flour, ripe bananas, and warm spices.
Preparation Time: 15 minutes
Cooking Time: 60 minutes
Total Time: 75 minutes
Servings: 8
Ingredients
2 cups gluten-free flour
1 teaspoon baking soda
1/2 teaspoon baking powder
1/2 teaspoon salt
1 teaspoon ground cinnamon
1/2 teaspoon ground nutmeg
3 ripe bananas, mashed
1/2 cup coconut sugar or brown sugar
1/4 cup coconut oil, melted
1/4 cup unsweetened applesauce
1 teaspoon vanilla extract
1/2 cup chopped walnuts or pecans (optional)
Instructions
1. Preheat oven to 350°F (175°C). Grease a 9x5 inch loaf pan or line with parchment paper.
2. In a large bowl, whisk together gluten-free flour, baking soda, baking powder, salt, cinnamon, and nutmeg.
3. In another bowl, mix mashed bananas, coconut sugar, melted coconut oil, applesauce, and vanilla extract until well combined.
4. Add wet ingredients to dry ingredients and stir until just combined. Fold in chopped nuts if using.
5. Pour batter into the prepared loaf pan and smooth the top with a spatula.
6. Bake for 55-60 minutes, or until a toothpick inserted into the center comes out clean.
7. Allow banana bread to cool in the pan for 10 minutes before transferring to a wire rack to cool completely.
Nutritional Info: Calories: 280, Protein: 5g, Carbohydrates: 35g, Fat: 12g, Fiber: 4g

Quinoa Breakfast Bowl

A hearty and nutritious breakfast bowl packed with protein, fiber, and flavor.
Preparation Time: 5 minutes
Cooking Time: 10 minutes (if cooking quinoa from scratch)
Total Time: 15 minutes
Ingredients
1 cup cooked quinoa
1/2 cup mixed berries
1 tablespoon almond butter

1 tablespoon maple syrup
1 tablespoon chopped nuts (e.g., almonds, walnuts)
Instructions
1. In a bowl, layer cooked quinoa with mixed berries.
2. Drizzle almond butter and maple syrup over the top.
3. Sprinkle with chopped nuts.
4. Serve immediately.
Nutritional Info: Calories: 350, Protein: 10g, Carbohydrates: 55g, Fat: 10g, Fiber: 8g

Vegan Gluten-Free Pancakes

Fluffy and delicious pancakes made without gluten or dairy.
Preparation Time: 10 minutes
Cooking Time: 15 minutes
Total Time: 25 minutes
Serving Time: Immediately
Ingredients:
1 cup gluten-free flour blend
1 tablespoon ground flaxseed mixed with 3 tablespoons water (as an egg substitute)
1 tablespoon maple syrup
1 teaspoon baking powder
1/2 teaspoon vanilla extract
1 cup almond milk
Coconut oil for cooking
Instructions
1. In a mixing bowl, whisk together the flour, baking powder, and flaxseed mixture.
2. Add maple syrup, vanilla extract, and almond milk. Mix until smooth.
3. Heat a skillet over medium heat and lightly grease with coconut oil.
4. Pour batter onto the skillet to form pancakes.
5. Cook until bubbles form on the surface, then flip and cook until golden brown on both sides.
6. Serve hot with your favorite toppings.
Nutritional Info: Calories: 250, Protein: 5g, Carbohydrates: 40g, Fat: 8g, Fiber: 4g

Coconut Rice Porridge

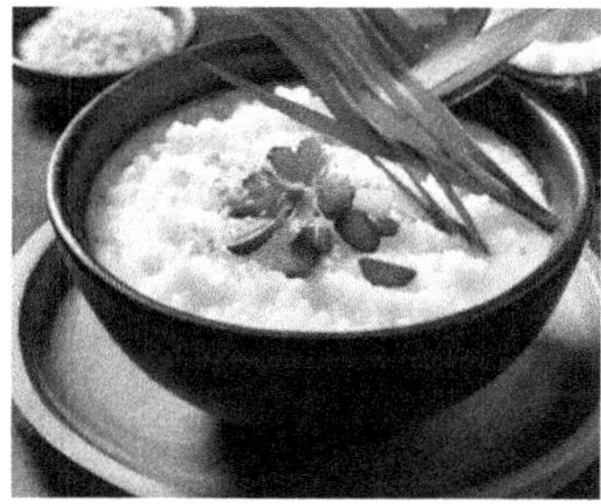

Creamy and comforting rice porridge flavored with coconut milk.

Preparation Time: 5 minutes
Cooking Time: 25 minutes
Total Time: 30 minutes
Servings: 2
Ingredients
1/2 cup white rice
1 cup coconut milk
1 cup water
2 tablespoons maple syrup
Pinch of salt
Toppings: sliced bananas, shredded coconut, chopped nuts
Instructions
1. Rinse the rice under cold water until the water runs clear.
2. In a saucepan, combine rice, coconut milk, water, maple syrup, and salt.
3. Bring to a boil, then reduce heat to low and simmer for 20-25 minutes, stirring occasionally, until rice is tender and creamy.
4. Serve hot with your favorite toppings.
Nutritional Info: Calories: 300, Protein: 4g, Carbohydrates: 45g, Fat: 12g, Fiber: 2g
Apple Cinnamon Oatmeal
Warm and comforting oatmeal flavored with apple and cinnamon.
Preparation Time: 5 minutes
Cooking Time: 10 minutes
Total Time: 15 minutes
Servings: 2
Ingredients
1 cup gluten-free rolled oats
2 cups almond milk or any plant-based milk
1 apple, peeled and diced
1 tablespoon maple syrup or sweetener of choice
1 teaspoon ground cinnamon
Pinch of salt
Toppings: sliced almonds, hemp seeds
Instructions
1. In a saucepan, combine oats, almond milk, diced apple, maple syrup, cinnamon, and salt.
2. Bring to a boil, then reduce heat to low and simmer for 7-10 minutes, stirring occasionally, until oats are cooked and creamy.
3. Serve hot with your favorite toppings.
Nutritional Info: Calories: 280, Protein: 8g, Carbohydrates: 45g, Fat: 6g, Fiber: 7g

Rice Flour Pancakes

Fluffy and tender pancakes made with rice flour.
Preparation Time: 10 minutes

Cooking Time: 10 minutes
Total Time: 20 minutes
Servings: 2

Ingredients

1 cup rice flour
1 tablespoon coconut sugar or sweetener of choice
1 teaspoon baking powder
Pinch of salt
1 cup almond milk
1 tablespoon coconut oil, melted
Optional toppings: sliced bananas, maple syrup

Instructions

1. In a bowl, whisk together rice flour, coconut sugar, baking powder, and salt.
2. Add almond milk and melted coconut oil, and stir until smooth.
3. Heat a non-stick skillet over medium heat and grease with little oil.
4. Pour 1/4 cup of batter onto the skillet for each pancake.
5. Cook the pancake until bubbles form on the surface, then flip and cook until golden brown.
6. Serve warm with your favorite toppings.

Nutritional Info: Calories: 320, Protein: 4g, Carbohydrates: 50g, Fat: 10g, Fiber: 2g

Banana Oatmeal Muffins

Moist and flavorful muffins made with gluten-free oats and ripe bananas.
Preparation Time: 10 minutes
Cooking Time: 20 minutes
Total Time: 30 minutes
Servings 6

Ingredients

1 cup gluten-free rolled oats
2 ripe bananas, mashed
1/4 cup almond milk
2 tablespoons maple syrup
1 teaspoon vanilla extract
1 teaspoon baking powder
Pinch of salt
Optional add-ins: chopped nuts, chocolate chips

Instructions

1. Preheat the oven to 350°F (175°C). Line a muffin tin with liners or lightly grease with coconut oil.
2. In a bowl, combine mashed bananas, almond milk, maple syrup, and vanilla extract.
3. Add gluten-free oats, baking powder, and salt, and stir until well combined.
4. Fold in any optional add-ins if desired.
5. Divide the batter equally among the muffin cups.
6. Bake the muffins until a toothpick inserted into the center comes out clean, for about 20 minutes.

7. Allow the muffins to cool before serving.
Nutritional Info: Calories: 180, Protein: 3g, Carbohydrates: 35g, Fat: 4g, Fiber: 4g

Chocolate Banana Overnight Oats

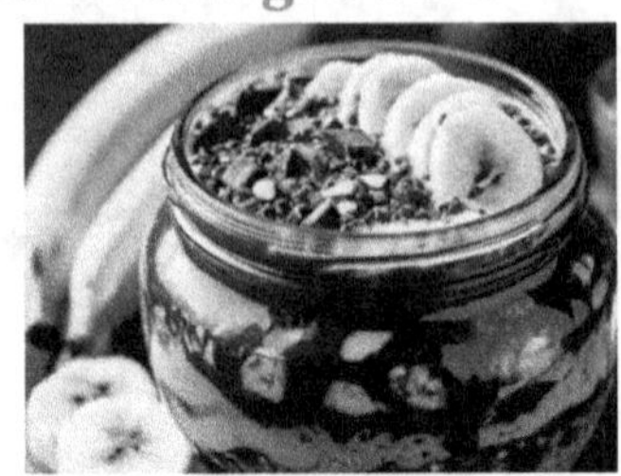

Creamy and indulgent overnight oats with chocolate and bananas.
Preparation Time: 5 minutes (plus chilling time)
Total Time: 8 hours 5 minutes
Servings: 2
Ingredients
1 cup gluten-free rolled oats
1 cup almond milk
2 tablespoons cocoa powder
2 tablespoons maple syrup
1 ripe banana, mashed
Optional toppings: sliced bananas, chocolate chips
Instructions
1. In a bowl, mix together oats, almond milk, cocoa powder, maple syrup, and mashed banana until well combined.
2. Divide the mixture into two jars or bowls.
3. Cover and refrigerate overnight or for at least 8 hours.
4. Before serving, top with sliced bananas and chocolate chips if desired.
Nutritional Info: Calories: 300, Protein: 6g, Carbohydrates: 50g, Fat: 8g, Fiber: 8g

Chia Seed Pudding

A creamy and nutritious pudding loaded with omega-3s and fiber.
Preparation Time: 5 minutes (plus chilling time)
Cooking Time: 0 minutes
Total Time: 5 minutes + chilling time (4 hours)
Serving Time: After chilling
Ingredients
1/4 cup chia seeds
1 cup almond milk
1 tablespoon maple syrup
Fresh fruit for topping
Instructions
1. In a bowl, mix chia seeds, almond milk, and maple syrup.
2. Stir well, then cover and refrigerate for at least 4 hours or overnight.
3. Before serving, stir the pudding again and top with fresh fruit.

Nutritional Info: Calories: 200, Protein: 6g, Carbohydrates: 20g, Fat: 10g, Fiber: 10g

Tofu Scramble

A savory and protein-packed alternative to scrambled eggs
Preparation Time: 10 minutes
Cooking Time: 10 minutes
Total Time: 20 minutes
Serving Time: Immediately
Ingredients:
1 block firm tofu, crumbled
1 tablespoon nutritional yeast
1/2 teaspoon turmeric
1/2 teaspoon garlic powder
Salt and pepper to taste
Mixed vegetables (e.g., bell peppers, onions, spinach)
Olive oil for cooking
Instructions
1. Heat olive oil in a skillet over medium heat.
2. Add mixed vegetables and cook until softened.
3. Add crumbled tofu, nutritional yeast, turmeric, garlic powder, salt, and pepper.
4. Cook for 5-7 minutes, stirring occasionally, until tofu is heated through and resembles scrambled   eggs.
5. Serve hot with toast or gluten-free tortillas.
Nutritional Info: Calories: 250, Protein: 20g, Carbohydrates: 10g, Fat: 15g, Fiber: 5g

Coconut Flour Banana Muffins

Moist and flavorful muffins made with coconut flour and ripe bananas.
Preparation Time: 10 minutes
Cooking Time: 20 minutes
Total Time: 30 minutes
Serving Time: Immediately
Ingredients
1 cup coconut flour
1 teaspoon baking powder
1/2 teaspoon baking soda
Pinch of salt
3 ripe bananas, mashed
1/4 cup maple syrup
1/4 cup almond milk
1/4 cup coconut oil, melted
1 teaspoon vanilla extract
Instructions
1. Preheat the oven to 350°F and properly line a muffin tin with paper liners.
2. In a large mixing bowl, whisk together coconut flour, baking soda, baking powder and salt.

3. In another mixing bowl, mix mashed bananas, maple syrup, almond milk, melted coconut oil, and vanilla extract.
4. Add wet ingredients to dry ingredients and stir until well combined.
5. Divide the batter evenly among the muffin cups.
6. Bake the muffins for about 20 minutes, or until a toothpick inserted into the center comes out clean.
7. Allow muffins to cool before serving.
Nutritional Info: Calories: 180, Protein: 3g, Carbohydrates: 25g, Fat: 8g, Fiber: 5g

Avocado Toast with Hemp Seeds

A simple yet satisfying breakfast featuring creamy avocado on gluten-free toast.
Preparation Time: 5 minutes
Cooking Time: 0 minutes
Total Time: 5 minutes
Serving Time: Immediately
Ingredients
2 slices gluten-free bread, toasted
1 ripe avocado, mashed
Hemp seeds for sprinkling
Salt and pepper to taste
Instructions
1. Toast gluten-free bread until golden brown.
2. Spread the mashed avocado evenly over the toast.
3. Sprinkle hemp seeds on top.
4. Season with salt and pepper to taste.
5. Serve immediately.
Nutritional Info: Calories: 250, Protein: 7g, Carbohydrates: 20g, Fat: 15g, Fiber: 10g

Berry Smoothie Bowl

A refreshing and vibrant smoothie bowl packed with antioxidants and vitamins.
Preparation Time: 5 minutes
Cooking Time: 0 minutes
Total Time: 5 minutes
Serving Time: Immediately
Ingredients
1 cup mixed berries (fresh or frozen)
1 ripe banana
1/2 cup almond milk
1 tablespoon chia seeds
Toppings: sliced banana, granola, shredded coconut
Instructions
1. In a blender, combine mixed berries, banana, almond milk, and chia seeds.
2. Blend until smooth and creamy.
3. Pour into a bowl and top with sliced banana, granola, and shredded coconut.
4. Serve immediately.
Nutritional Info: Calories: 300, Protein: 5g, Carbohydrates: 45g, Fat: 10g, Fiber: 12g

Sweet Potato Breakfast Hash

A savory and satisfying breakfast hash made with sweet potatoes and vegetables.
Preparation Time: 10 minutes
Cooking Time: 20 minutes
Total Time: 30 minutes
Serving Time: Immediately

Ingredients
2 medium sweet potatoes, diced
1 bell pepper, diced
1 onion, diced
2 cloves garlic, minced
1 teaspoon paprika
1/2 teaspoon cumin
Salt and pepper to taste
Olive oil for cooking

Instructions
1. Heat olive oil in a skillet over medium heat.
2. Add diced sweet potatoes and cook until slightly softened.
3. Add diced bell pepper, onion, and minced garlic.
4. Season with paprika, cumin, salt, and pepper.
5. Cook until vegetables are tender and lightly browned.
6. Serve hot as is or with a side of avocado slices.
Nutritional Info: Calories: 280, Protein: 4g, Carbohydrates: 45g, Fat: 8g, Fiber: 8g

Kale mango Smoothie

A nutritious and energizing smoothie packed with leafy greens and fruits.
Preparation Time: 5 minutes
Cooking Time: 0 minutes
Total Time: 5 minutes
Serving Time: Immediately

Ingredients
2 cups kale
1 ripe banana
1/2 cup frozen mango chunks
1/2 cup pineapple chunks
1 tablespoon chia seeds
1 cup coconut water or almond milk

Instructions
1. In a blender, combine spinach or kale, banana, mango chunks, pineapple chunks, chia seeds, and coconut water or almond milk.
2. Blend until smooth and creamy.
3. Pour into a serving glass and serve immediately.
Nutritional Info: Calories: 250, Protein: 5g, Carbohydrates: 45g, Fat: 5g, Fiber: 10g

Overnight Oats

A convenient and customizable breakfast option that's ready to eat in the morning.
Preparation Time: 5 minutes
Cooking Time: 0 minutes
Total Time: Overnight (at least 4 hours)
Serving Time: After chilling
Ingredients
1/2 cup gluten-free rolled oats
1/2 cup almond milk
1 tablespoon maple syrup
1 tablespoon chia seeds
Toppings: sliced banana, berries, nuts, shredded coconut
Instructions
1. In a jar or container, combine rolled oats, almond milk, maple syrup, and chia seeds.
2. Stir well, then cover and refrigerate overnight or for at least 4 hours.
3. In the morning, give the oats a good stir and add your favorite toppings before serving.
Nutritional Info: Calories: 300, Protein: 7g, Carbohydrates: 50g, Fat: 8g, Fiber: 10g

Almond Flour Pancakes with Blueberry Compote

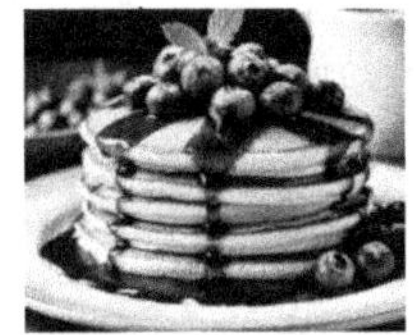

Fluffy pancakes made with almond flour, topped with a sweet and tangy blueberry compote.
Preparation Time: 10 minutes
Cooking Time: 10 minutes
Total Time: 20 minutes
Servings: 2
Ingredients
1 cup almond flour
2 tablespoons ground flaxseed
1 teaspoon baking powder
1 ripe banana, mashed
1/2 cup almond milk
1 teaspoon vanilla extract
1 cup fresh or frozen blueberries
Instructions
1. In a mixing bowl, combine ground flaxseed, almond flour and baking powder.
2. Add mashed banana, almond milk, and vanilla extract. Mix until well combined.
3. Heat a non-stick pan over medium heat. Pour 1/4 cup of batter onto the pan for each pancake.
4. Cook until bubbles form on the surface, then flip and cook until golden brown.

5. In a small saucepan, heat blueberries until they release their juices and slightly thicken.
6. Serve pancakes topped with blueberry compote.
Nutritional Info: Calories: 280, Protein: 8g, Fat: 16g, Carbohydrates: 29g, Fiber: 7g

Quinoa Breakfast Bowl with Avocado and Nuts

Nutrient-packed quinoa bowl topped with creamy avocado and crunchy nuts.
Preparation Time: 5 minutes
Cooking Time: 15 minutes (for quinoa)
Total Time: 20 minutes
Serving: 1
Ingredients
1 cup cooked quinoa
1 ripe avocado, sliced
1/4 cup mixed nuts (almonds, walnuts, pecans)
1 tablespoon maple syrup
Pinch of cinnamon
Instructions
1. Cook quinoa according to package instructions.
2. In a bowl, layer cooked quinoa, sliced avocado, and mixed nuts.
3. Drizzle with maple syrup and sprinkle with cinnamon.
4. Serve immediately.
Nutritional Info: Calories: 480, Protein: 12g, Fat: 29g, Carbohydrates: 45g, Fiber: 10g

Avocado Toast with Almond Butter and Chia Seeds

Creamy avocado spread on gluten-free toast, topped with almond butter and chia seeds for added protein and omega-3s.
Preparation Time: 5 minutes
Cooking Time: N/A
Total Time: 5 minutes
Serving: 1
Ingredients
 2 slices gluten-free bread
1 ripe avocado, mashed
2 tablespoons almond butter
1 tablespoon chia seeds
Pinch of sea salt
Instructions
1. Toast gluten-free bread until golden brown.
2. Spread the mashed avocado evenly over the toast.
3. Drizzle almond butter on top and sprinkle with chia seeds.
4. Season with a pinch of sea salt.
5. Serve immediately.
Nutritional Info: Calories: 380, Protein: 12g, Fat: 25g, Carbohydrates: 32g, Fiber: 15g

Almond Flour Banana Bread

Moist and flavorful banana bread made with almond flour, perfect for a gluten-free breakfast treat.
Preparation Time: 10 minutes
Cooking Time: 45 minutes
Total Time: 55 minutes
Servings: 8
Ingredients
2 ripe bananas, mashed
2 cups almond flour
1/4 cup coconut sugar
1/4 cup almond milk
2 tablespoons coconut oil, melted
1 teaspoon vanilla extract
1 teaspoon baking powder
Pinch of salt
Instructions
1. Preheat oven to 350°F (175°C).
2. Grease a loaf pan with coconut oil.
3. In a large mixing bowl, combine mashed bananas, almond flour, coconut sugar, almond milk, melted coconut oil, vanilla extract, baking powder, and salt.
4. Mix until well combined.
5. Pour the batter into the prepared loaf pan.
6. Bake for 40-45 minutes, or until a toothpick inserted into the center comes out clean.
7. Allow the banana bread to cool before slicing and serving.
Nutritional Info: Calories: 280, Protein: 7g, Fat: 20g, Carbohydrates: 22g, Fiber: 5g

Quinoa Breakfast Cookies

Soft and chewy breakfast cookies made with quinoa, almond flour, and dried fruits.
Preparation Time: 10 minutes
Cooking Time: 15 minutes
Total Time: 25 minutes
Servings: 6
Ingredients
1 cup cooked quinoa
1 cup almond flour
1/4 cup maple syrup
1/4 cup dried cranberries
1/4 cup chopped almonds
1/4 cup shredded coconut
1 teaspoon vanilla extract
1/2 teaspoon cinnamon
Pinch of salt
Instructions
1. Preheat oven to 350°F (175°C).

2. Line a baking sheet with parchment paper.

3. In a mixing bowl, combine cooked quinoa, almond flour, maple syrup, dried cranberries, chopped almonds, shredded coconut, vanilla extract, cinnamon, and salt.

4. Mix until well combined.

5. Scoop spoonfuls of the dough onto the prepared baking sheet, flattening slightly with your fingers.

6. Bake the cookie for 12-15 minutes, or until golden brown.

7. Allow the cookies to cool on the baking sheet before serving.

Nutritional Info: Calories: 260, Protein: 6g, Fat: 15g, Carbohydrates: 27g, Fiber: 4g

Avocado and Spinach Smoothie Bowl

Creamy green smoothie bowl packed with avocado, spinach, and nuts for a nutritious breakfast.

Preparation Time: 5 minutes

Cooking Time: N/A

Total Time: 5 minutes

Servings: 1

Ingredients

1 ripe avocado

2 cups fresh spinach

1 frozen banana

1/2 cup almond milk

2 tablespoons almond butter

1 tablespoon chia seeds

Handful of mixed nuts (walnuts, almonds, cashews)

Instructions

1. In a blender, combine ripe avocado, fresh spinach, frozen banana, almond milk, and almond butter.

   Blend until smooth.

2. Pour the smoothie into a bowl.

3. Top with chia seeds and mixed nuts.

4. Serve immediately with a spoon.

Nutritional Info: Calories: 450, Protein: 12g, Fat: 32g, Carbohydrates: 38g, Fiber: 14g

Almond Flour Waffles

Crispy gluten-free waffles made with almond flour, perfect for a weekend breakfast.

Preparation Time: 10 minutes

Cooking Time: 10 minutes

Total Time: 20 minutes

Servings: 4

Ingredients

1 1/2 cups almond flour

2 tablespoons coconut flour

1 teaspoon baking powder

1/4 teaspoon salt

2 tablespoons maple syrup

2 tablespoons coconut oil, melted
3/4 cup almond milk
1 teaspoon vanilla extract
Instructions
1. Preheat waffle iron according to manufacturer's instructions.
2. In a mixing medium bowl, combine the almond flour, baking powder, coconut flour and salt.
3. In a separate bowl, whisk together maple syrup, melted coconut oil, almond milk, and vanilla extract.
4. Combine the wet ingredients with the dry ingredients and mix until smooth.
5. Grease the waffle iron with coconut oil and pour in the batter.
6. Cook according to the waffle iron instructions, until golden and crispy.
7. Serve warm with your favorite toppings.
Nutritional Info (without toppings): Calories: 320, Protein: 10g, Fat: 25g, Carbohydrates:20g, Fiber

Quinoa Breakfast Porridge with Almond Milk

Warm and comforting quinoa porridge made with almond milk, topped with fresh fruit and nuts.
Preparation Time: 5 minutes
Cooking Time: 20 minutes
Total Time: 25 minutes
Servings: 2
Ingredients
1/2 cup quinoa, rinsed
1 cup almond milk
1 tablespoon maple syrup
1/2 teaspoon cinnamon
Pinch of salt
Fresh fruit (berries, sliced banana)
Mixed nuts (almonds, walnuts, pecans)
Instructions
1. In a saucepan, combine quinoa, almond milk, maple syrup, cinnamon, and salt.
2. Bring to a boil, then reduce heat to low and simmer for 15-20 minutes, or until quinoa is tender and the mixture has thickened.
3. Serve the quinoa porridge in bowls, topped with fresh fruit and mixed nuts.
4. Drizzle with additional maple syrup if desired.
Nutritional Info: Calories: 280, Protein: 8g, Fat: 12g, Carbohydrates: 35g, Fiber: 6g

Avocado Breakfast Burrito with Almond Flour Tortilla

Hearty breakfast burrito filled with creamy avocado, scrambled tofu, and veggies, wrapped in a homemade almond flour tortilla.
Preparation Time: 15 minutes
Cooking Time: 15 minutes
Total Time: 30 minutes
Servings: 2
Ingredients

For the almond flour tortillas:
1 cup almond flour
2 tablespoons ground flaxseed
1/4 teaspoon salt
1/4 cup warm water
For the filling:
1 ripe avocado, sliced
1/2 cup scrambled tofu
1/4 cup diced tomatoes
1/4 cup diced bell peppers
Handful of spinach leaves
Hot sauce (optional)

Instructions

1. To make the almond flour tortillas, combine almond flour, ground flaxseed, and salt in a mixing bowl.
2. Gradually add warm water and knead until a dough forms.
3. Properly divide the dough into 4 even portions and roll out each portion into a very thin tortilla.
4. Cook the tortillas in a heated skillet for 1-2 minutes on each side, until lightly golden brown.
5. To assemble the burritos, place sliced avocado, scrambled tofu, diced tomatoes, diced bell peppers, and spinach leaves in the center of each tortilla.
6. Drizzle with hot sauce if desired.
7. Roll up the tortillas, tucking in the sides, to form burritos.
8. Serve immediately.

Nutritional Info: Calories: 420, Protein: 15g, Fat: 32g, Carbohydrates: 24g, Fiber: 12g

Nutty Almond Butter Smoothie

Creamy and satisfying smoothie packed with almond butter, banana, and nuts for a protein-rich breakfast.

Preparation Time: 5 minutes
Cooking Time: N/A
Total Time: 5 minutes
Serving: 1

Ingredients

1 ripe banana
2 tablespoons almond butter
1 cup almond milk
1 tablespoon chia seeds
Handful of mixed nuts (almonds, walnuts, cashews)
Ice cubes (optional)

Instructions

1. In a blender, combine ripe banana, almond butter, almond milk, chia seeds, and ice cubes (if using).
2. Blend until smooth and creamy.
3. Pour the smoothie into a glass.

4. Garnish with a handful of mixed nuts.
5. Serve immediately with a straw.
Nutritional Info: Calories: 380, Protein: 10g, Fat: 28g, Carbohydrates: 30g, Fiber: 8g

Lunch Recipes

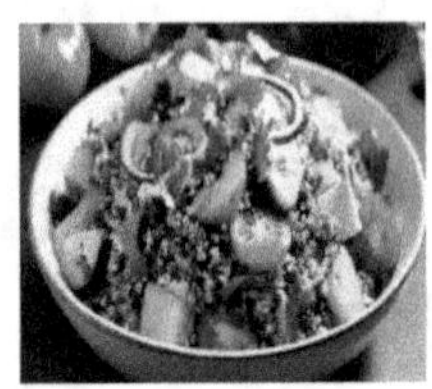

Quinoa Salad with Roasted Vegetables

A colorful and nutritious salad packed with protein-rich quinoa and flavorful roasted vegetables.
Preparation Time: 10 minutes
Cooking Time: 25 minutes
Total Time: 35 minutes
Servings: 4
Ingredients
1 cup quinoa
Assorted vegetables (such as bell peppers, cherry tomatoes, zucchini)
Olive oil
Salt and pepper to taste
Fresh herbs (optional)
Instructions
1. Preheat oven to 400°F (200°C).
2. Cook quinoa according to package instructions.
3. Chop vegetables and toss with olive oil, salt, and pepper. Roast in the preheated oven for 20-25 minutes.
4. Once quinoa and vegetables are cooked, mix them together in a large bowl.
5. Garnish with fresh herbs if desired. Serve warm or cold.
Nutritional Info: Calories: 250, Protein: 8g, Fat: 6g, Carbohydrates: 40g, Fiber: 6g

Sweet Potato and Black Bean Tacos

A hearty and satisfying taco filling made with sweet potatoes and black beans, served in gluten-free corn tortillas.
Preparation Time: 10 minutes
Cooking Time: 20 minutes
Total Time: 30 minutes
Servings: 4
Ingredients
2 medium sweet potatoes, diced
1 can black beans, drained and rinsed

1 teaspoon cumin
1 teaspoon chili powder
Salt and pepper to taste
Corn tortillas
Toppings of choice (avocado, salsa, cilantro)
Instructions
1. In a skillet, sauté diced sweet potatoes until tender.
2. Add black beans, cumin, chili powder, salt, and pepper. Cook for an additional 5-7 minutes.
3. Warm corn tortillas in a separate skillet or microwave.
4. Fill tortillas with the sweet potato and black bean mixture.
5. Top with desired toppings such as avocado, salsa, and cilantro.
Nutritional Info: Calories: 300, Protein: 8g, Fat: 3g, Carbohydrates: 60g, Fiber: 10g

Spinach and Mushroom Quiche

A savory quiche filled with spinach, mushrooms, and dairy-free cheese, all nestled in a gluten-free crust.

Preparation Time: 15 minutes
Cooking Time: 40 minutes
Total Time: 55 minutes
Servings: 6
Ingredients
1 gluten-free pie crust (store-bought or homemade)
2 cups fresh spinach, chopped
1 cup mushrooms, sliced
1 onion, diced
1 cup dairy-free cheese, shredded
4 eggs
1 cup almond milk
Salt and pepper to taste
Instructions
1. Preheat oven to 375°F (190°C).
2. In a skillet, sauté onions until translucent. Add mushrooms and spinach, and cook until softened.
3. In a bowl, whisk together eggs, almond milk, salt, and pepper.
4. Place the cooked vegetables and dairy-free cheese into the pie crust.
5. Pour the egg mixture over the vegetables and cheese.
6. Bake for 35-40 minutes or until the quiche is set and golden brown.
Nutritional Info: Calories: 250, Protein: 10g, Fat: 15g, Carbohydrates: 20g, Fiber: 3g

Zucchini Noodles with Pesto

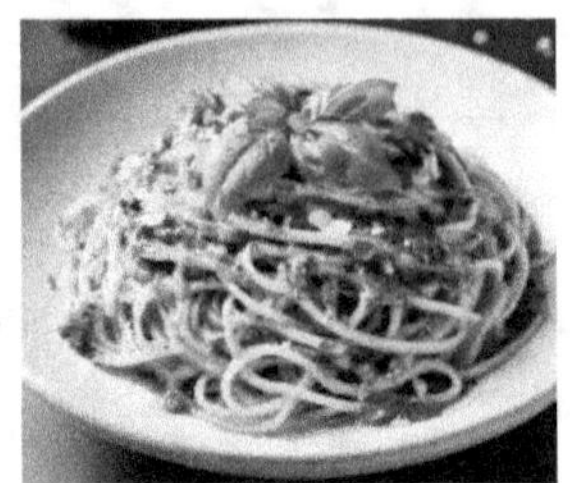

A light and refreshing dish made with zucchini noodles and homemade dairy-free pesto sauce.
Preparation Time: 15 minutes
Cooking Time: 0 minutes
Total Time: 15 minutes
Servings: 4
Ingredients
4 medium zucchini, spiralized into noodles
1 cup fresh basil leaves
1/4 cup pine nuts
2 cloves garlic
1/4 cup nutritional yeast
1/4 cup olive oil
Salt and pepper to taste
Instructions
1. In a food processor, combine basil, pine nuts, garlic, nutritional yeast, olive oil, salt, and pepper. Blend until smooth to make the pesto sauce.
2. Spiralize zucchini into noodles using a spiralizer or julienne peeler.
3. Toss the zucchini noodles with the pesto sauce until evenly coated.
4. Serve immediately, garnished with additional pine nuts or basil if desired.
Nutritional Info: Calories: 200, Protein: 5g, Fat: 15g, Carbohydrates: 10g, Fiber: 4g

Chickpea Salad Sandwich

A satisfying sandwich filling made with mashed chickpeas, crunchy vegetables, and dairy-free mayo.
Preparation Time: 10 minutes
Cooking Time: 0 minutes
Total Time: 10 minutes
Servings: 2
Ingredients
1 can chickpeas, drained and rinsed
1/4 cup dairy-free mayo
1/4 cup celery, diced
1/4 cup red bell pepper, diced
2 tablespoons red onion, finely chopped
1 tablespoon lemon juice
Salt and pepper to taste
Gluten-free bread slices

Lettuce leaves and tomato slices for serving
Instructions
1. In a medium mixing bowl, mash the chickpeas with a potato masher or fork.
2. Add dairy-free mayo, celery, bell pepper, red onion, lemon juice, salt, and pepper. Stir until well combined.
3. Toast gluten-free bread slices if desired.
4. Spread the chickpea salad mixture onto bread slices.
5. Top with lettuce leaves, tomato slices, and another slice of bread to make sandwiches.
Nutritional Info: Calories: 300, Protein: 10g, Fat: 10g, Carbohydrates: 40g, Fiber: 10g

Cauliflower Rice Stir-Fry

A low-carb alternative to traditional rice, cauliflower rice is stir-fried with colorful vegetables and tofu.
Preparation Time: 15 minutes
Cooking Time: 15 minutes
Total Time: 30 minutes
Servings: 4
Ingredients
1 head cauliflower, grated into rice-like pieces
1 cup mixed vegetables (broccoli, bell peppers, snap peas and more)
1 block tofu, pressed and cubed
2 tablespoons tamari or soy sauce
1 tablespoon sesame oil
2 cloves garlic, minced
1 teaspoon ginger, grated
Green onions for garnish
Instructions
1. In a large skillet or wok, heat sesame oil over medium heat.
2. Add minced garlic and grated ginger, and sauté for 1-2 minutes.
3. Add cubed tofu and cook until browned on all sides.
4. Push tofu to one side of the skillet and add mixed vegetables. Stir-fry until tender-crisp.
5. Push vegetables to the side and add cauliflower rice to the skillet. Cook for 3-5 minutes, stirring occasionally.
6. Mix everything together, then add tamari or soy sauce. Stir well to combine.
7. Garnish the cauliflower rice stir-fry with sliced green onions before serving. Enjoy!
Nutritional Info: Calories: 200, Protein: 15g, Fat: 8g, Carbohydrates: 20g, Fiber: 8g

Avocado and White Bean Salad

A creamy and protein-packed salad featuring avocado, white beans, and a zesty lime dressing.
Preparation Time: 10 minutes
Cooking Time: 0 minutes
Total Time: 10 minutes
Servings: 4

Ingredients
2 ripe avocados, diced
1 can white beans, drained and rinsed
1 bell pepper, diced
1/4 cup red onion, finely chopped
Juice of 2 limes
2 tablespoons olive oil
1 tablespoon fresh cilantro, chopped
Salt and pepper to taste
Instructions
1. In a large bowl, combine diced avocados, white beans, bell pepper, and red onion.
2. In a small bowl, whisk together lime juice, olive oil, cilantro, salt, and pepper to make the dressing.
3. Pour the dressing over the salad ingredients and toss gently to coat.
4. Serve immediately, or refrigerate until ready to serve.
Nutritional Info: Calories: 250, Protein: 8g, Fat: 15g, Carbohydrates: 25g, Fiber: 10g

Vegetable Stir-Fry with Brown Rice

Colorful stir-fried vegetables served over nutty brown rice, seasoned with a savory sauce.
Preparation Time: 15 minutes
Cooking Time: 20 minutes
Total Time: 35 minutes
Servings: 4
Ingredients
1 cup brown rice
2 cups water
2 tablespoons sesame oil
2 cups mixed vegetables (bell peppers, carrots, snap peas, broccoli and more)
3 cloves garlic, minced
1 tablespoon grated ginger
1/4 cup tamari or soy sauce
1 tablespoon rice vinegar
1 tablespoon maple syrup
Sesame seeds for garnish
Instructions
1. In a saucepan, bring drinkable water to a boil.
2. Add brown rice. Cover the saucepan and then let it simmer for about 40 minutes, or until tender.
3. Heat sesame oil in a large skillet over medium heat.
4. Add garlic and ginger, cook until fragrant.
5. Add mixed vegetables to the skillet, stir-fry until tender.
6. In a small bowl, mix tamari or soy sauce, rice vinegar, and maple syrup.
7. Pour over the vegetables and cook for 2-3 minutes.
8. Serve the stir-fried vegetables over cooked brown rice, garnished with sesame seeds.

Nutritional Info: Calories: 280, Protein: 8g, Carbohydrates: 45g, Fat: 6g, Fiber: 8g

Quinoa Salad with Avocado and Chickpeas

A refreshing salad featuring protein-packed quinoa, creamy avocado, crunchy vegetables, and chickpeas, tossed in a tangy vinaigrette.
Preparation Time: 15 minutes
Cooking Time: 15 minutes
Total Time: 30 minutes
Servings: 4
Ingredients
1 cup quinoa, rinsed
2 cups water or vegetable broth
1 avocado, diced
1 can chickpeas, drained and rinsed
1 cup cherry tomatoes, halved
1/2 cucumber, diced
1/4 cup red onion, diced
1/4 cup fresh cilantro, chopped
Juice of 1 lemon
2 tablespoons olive oil
Salt and pepper to taste
Instructions
1. In a medium saucepan, bring drinkable water or vegetable broth to a boil.
2. Add quinoa, cover, and simmer for 15 minutes, or until cooked.
3. Let it cool.
4. In a large bowl, combine cooked quinoa, diced avocado, chickpeas, cherry tomatoes, cucumber, red onion, and cilantro.
5. In a small bowl, whisk together lemon juice, olive oil, salt, and pepper.
6. Pour over the salad and toss to coat.
7. Serve chilled or at room temperature.
Nutritional Info: Calories: 320, Protein: 10g, Carbohydrates: 45g, Fat: 12g, Fiber: 10g

Gluten-Free Veggie Wrap with Hummus

A nutritious and filling wrap filled with a variety of fresh vegetables and creamy hummus, wrapped in a gluten-free tortilla.
Preparation Time: 10 minutes
Cooking Time: 0 minutes
Total Time: 10 minutes
Serving Size: 2
Ingredients
2 gluten-free tortillas
1/2 cup hummus
1/2 cup mixed salad greens
1/2 cup shredded carrots
1/2 cup cucumber slices
1/2 cup bell pepper strips

1/4 cup red cabbage, shredded

1/4 cup alfalfa sprouts

Instructions

1. Lay out the gluten-free tortillas on a clean surface.

2. Spread hummus evenly over each tortilla.

3. Layer mixed salad greens, shredded carrots, cucumber slices, bell pepper strips, red cabbage, and alfalfa sprouts on top of the hummus.

4. Roll up the tortillas tightly.

5. Cut each wrap in half and serve immediately.

Nutritional Info: Calories: 280, Protein: 8g, Carbohydrates: 40g, Fat: 10g, Fiber: 8g

Rainbow Quinoa Salad with Citrus Dressing

A vibrant and refreshing salad featuring a rainbow of vegetables, protein-rich quinoa, and a tangy citrus dressing.

Preparation Time: 20 minutes

Cooking Time: 15 minutes

Total Time: 35 minutes

Servings: 4

Ingredients

1 cup quinoa, rinsed

2 cups water or vegetable broth

1 cup cherry tomatoes, halved

1/2 cup shredded carrots

1/2 cup diced bell peppers (red, yellow, or orange)

1/2 cup diced cucumber

1/4 cup diced red onion

1/4 cup chopped fresh parsley

Juice of 2 oranges

Juice of 1 lemon

2 tablespoons olive oil

Salt and pepper to taste

Instructions

1. In a medium saucepan, bring drinkable water or vegetable broth to a boil.

2. Add quinoa, cover, and simmer for 15 minutes, or until cooked.

3. Let it cool.

4. In a large bowl, combine cooked quinoa, cherry tomatoes, shredded carrots, diced bell peppers, cucumber, red onion, and chopped parsley.

5. In a small bowl, whisk together orange juice, lemon juice, olive oil, salt, and pepper to make the dressing.

6. Pour the dressing on the salad and toss until coaedt.

7. Serve chilled or at room temperature.

Nutritional Info: Calories: 290, Protein: 8g, Carbohydrates: 45g, Fat: 8g, Fiber: 8g

Veggie Quinoa Bowl with Tahini Dressing

A nourishing bowl featuring quinoa, roasted vegetables, avocado, and a creamy tahini dressing.

Preparation Time: 20 minutes

Cooking Time: 25 minutes
Total Time: 45 minutes
Servings: 4
Ingredients
1 cup quinoa, rinsed
2 cups water or vegetable broth
2 cups mixed vegetables (bell peppers, zucchini, eggplant, cherry tomatoes)
2 tablespoons olive oil
1 teaspoon dried oregano
Salt and pepper to taste
1 avocado, sliced
1/4 cup tahini
Juice of 1 lemon
2 tablespoons water
1 clove garlic, minced
Instructions
1. In a saucepan, bring vegetable broth or drinkable water to a boil.
2. Add quinoa, cover, and simmer for 15 minutes, or until cooked.
3. Let it cool.
4. Preheat oven to 400°F (200°C).
5. Place mixed vegetables on a baking sheet, drizzle with olive oil, and sprinkle with dried oregano, salt, and pepper. Roast for about 25 minutes, or until tender.
6. In a small bowl, whisk together tahini, lemon juice, water, minced garlic, salt, and pepper to make the dressing.
7. To assemble the bowls, divide cooked quinoa among serving bowls.
8. Top with roasted vegetables and sliced avocado.
9. Drizzle tahini dressing over the bowls before serving.
Nutritional Info: Calories: 320, Protein: 10g, Carbohydrates: 45g, Fat: 12g, Fiber: 10g

Rainbow Veggie Salad with Lemon-Tahini Dressing

This vibrant salad combines a variety of colorful vegetables with a zesty lemon-tahini dressing for a refreshing and nutritious lunch option.
Preparation Time: 15 minutes
Cooking Time: 0 minutes
Total Time: 15 minutes
Servings: 2
Ingredients
2 cups mixed salad greens
1 medium cucumber, sliced
1 medium bell pepper, thinly sliced
1 medium carrot, grated
1/2 cup cherry tomatoes, halved
1/4 cup sliced red onion
2 tablespoons tahini
2 tablespoons fresh lemon juice
1 tablespoon olive oil

1 clove garlic, minced
Salt and pepper to taste
Instructions
1. In a large bowl, combine the mixed salad greens, cucumber slices, bell pepper slices, grated carrot, cherry tomatoes, and sliced red onion.
2. In a small bowl, whisk together the tahini, fresh lemon juice, olive oil, minced garlic, salt, and pepper to make the dressing.
3. Drizzle the dressing over the rainbow veggies salad and toss gently to coat.
4. Divide the salad between two plates and serve immediately.
Nutritional Info: Calories: 180, Protein: 4g, Carbohydrates: 14g, Fat: 13g, Fiber: 4g

Chickpea and Spinach Coconut Curry

This creamy coconut curry is packed with chickpeas, spinach, and aromatic spices, creating a flavorful and comforting lunch option.
Preparation Time: 15 minutes
Cooking Time: 25 minutes
Total Time: 40 minutes
Servings: 4
Ingredients
1 tablespoon coconut oil
1 onion, diced
3 cloves garlic, minced
1 tablespoon grated ginger
1 teaspoon ground cumin
1 teaspoon ground coriander
1/2 teaspoon turmeric
1/4 teaspoon cayenne pepper (optional)
1 can chickpeas, drained and rinsed
1 can full-fat coconut milk
2 cups baby spinach
Salt and pepper to taste
Cooked rice or quinoa for serving
Instructions
1. Heat oil in a large skillet over medium-high heat.
2. Add the onion and cook until softened.
3. Add minced garlic, grated ginger, ground cumin, ground coriander, turmeric, and cayenne pepper (if using).
4. Cook for 1-2 minutes, until fragrant.
5. Stir in chickpeas and full-fat coconut milk.
6. Simmer for 15 minutes, allowing the flavors to meld.
7. Add baby spinach to the skillet and cook until wilted.
8. Season with salt and pepper to taste.
9. Serve the curry hot over cooked rice or quinoa.
Nutritional Info: Calories: 320, Protein: 10g, Carbohydrates: 30g, Fat: 20g, Fiber: 8g

Mediterranean Quinoa Bowl

This Mediterranean-inspired quinoa bowl features a colorful array of vegetables, olives, and a tangy tahini dressing, providing a satisfying and nutritious lunch option.

Preparation Time: 20 minutes
Cooking Time: 15 minutes
Total Time: 35 minutes
Servings: 2

Ingredients

1 cup quinoa, rinsed
2 cups vegetable broth
1 cup cherry tomatoes, halved
1 cucumber, diced
1/4 cup Kalamata olives, pitted and halved
1/4 cup diced red onion
2 tablespoons chopped fresh parsley
2 tablespoons chopped fresh mint
2 tablespoons tahini
2 tablespoons fresh lemon juice
1 tablespoon olive oil
1 clove garlic, minced
Salt and pepper to taste

Instructions

1. In a medium saucepan, bring the vegetable broth to a boil over medium-high heat.
2. Add quinoa, reduce heat to low, cover, and simmer for 15 minutes, or until quinoa is cooked and broth is absorbed.
3. Remove from heat and let it sit for 5 minutes, then fluff with a fork.
4. In a large bowl, combine cooked quinoa, cherry tomatoes, diced cucumber, Kalamata olives, diced red onion, chopped fresh parsley, and chopped fresh mint.
5. In a small bowl, whisk together tahini, fresh lemon juice, olive oil, minced garlic, salt, and pepper to make the dressing.
6. Drizzle the dressing over the quinoa mixture and toss gently to coat.
7. Divide the quinoa mixture between two bowls and serve immediately.

Nutritional Info: Calories: 380, Protein: 10g, Carbohydrates: 45g, Fat: 18g, Fiber: 7g

Chickpea Avocado Salad Wraps

These refreshing salad wraps are filled with a creamy chickpea avocado salad and wrapped in lettuce leaves, providing a light and nutritious lunch option.

Preparation Time: 15 minutes
Cooking Time: 0 minutes
Total Time: 15 minutes
Servings: 4

Ingredients

1 can chickpeas, drained and rinsed
1 ripe avocado, mashed
1/4 cup diced red onion

1/4 cup chopped fresh cilantro
2 tablespoons lime juice
Salt and pepper to taste
8 large lettuce leaves (such as butter lettuce or romaine)
Instructions
1. In a medium bowl, combine chickpeas, mashed avocado, diced red onion, chopped fresh cilantro, lime juice, salt, and pepper.
2. Mash the chickpeas slightly with a fork while mixing.
3. Place a spoonful of the chickpea avocado salad onto each lettuce leaf.
4. Roll up the lettuce leaves to form wraps.
5. Serve immediately.
Nutritional Info: Calories: 200, Protein: 8g, Carbohydrates: 25g, Fat: 8g, Fiber: 10g
Tofu Stir-Fry with Mixed Vegetables

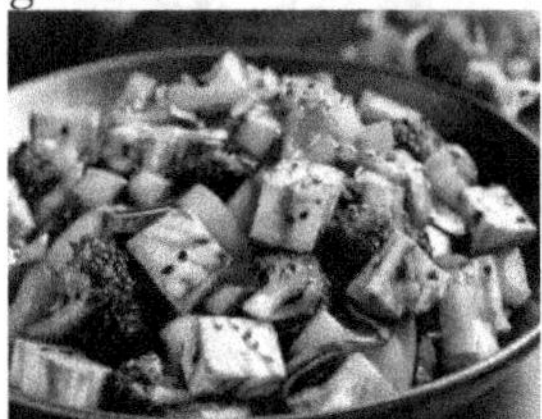

This colorful tofu stir-fry features a variety of mixed vegetables and savory tofu, making it a flavorful and satisfying lunch option.
Preparation Time: 15 minutes
Cooking Time: 15 minutes
Total Time: 30 minutes
Servings: 4
Ingredients
1 block firm tofu, drained and cubed
2 tablespoons tamari or soy sauce
1 tablespoon sesame oil
1 tablespoon olive oil
2 cloves garlic, minced
1 bell pepper, sliced
1 cup broccoli florets
1 carrot, julienned
1/2 cup snap peas
Cooked rice or quinoa for serving
Instructions
1. In a bowl, toss cubed tofu with tamari or soy sauce and sesame oil until evenly coated. Let marinate for 10 minutes.
2. Heat the oil in a large skillet over medium-high heat.
3. Add the garlic and cook until fragrant.
4. Add tofu to the skillet and cook until golden brown on all sides.
5. Remove tofu from the skillet and set aside.
6. In the same skillet, add sliced bell pepper, broccoli florets, julienned carrot, and snap peas.
7. Stir-fry until vegetables are tender-crisp.

8. Return the tofu to the skillet and toss to combine with the vegetables.
9. Serve the stir-fry hot over cooked rice or quinoa.
Nutritional Info: Calories: 220, Protein: 12g, Carbohydrates: 15g, Fat: 12g, Fiber: 6g

Cauliflower Rice Sushi Rolls

These sushi rolls are made with cauliflower rice instead of traditional rice, filled with colorful vegetables and avocado, making them a healthy and gluten-free lunch option.
Preparation Time: 30 minutes
Cooking Time: 15 minutes
Total Time: 45 minutes
Servings: 4
Ingredients
1 small head cauliflower
2 tablespoons rice vinegar
1 tablespoon maple syrup
1/2 teaspoon salt
4 nori sheets
1/2 cucumber, julienned
1 carrot, julienned
1/2 avocado, sliced
Pickled ginger and wasabi for serving (optional)
Instructions
1. Cut the cauliflower into florets and pulse in a food processor until it resembles rice.
2. In a small bowl, whisk together rice vinegar, maple syrup, and salt.
3. Pour over the cauliflower rice and mix well.
4. Place a nori sheet on a bamboo sushi mat or clean kitchen towel.
5. Spread a thin layer of cauliflower rice over the nori sheet, make sure you leave a small border around the edges.
6. Arrange cucumber, carrot, and avocado slices in a line across the bottom third of the nori sheet.
7. starting from the bottom, roll the nori sheet tightly into a cylinder, using the sushi mat or towel to help.
8. Repeat with the remaining nori sheets and fillings.
9. Use a sharp knife to slice each roll into about 7 or more pieces.
10. Serve sushi rolls with pickled ginger and wasabi, if desired.
Nutritional Info: Calories: 180, Protein: 6g, Carbohydrates: 25g, Fat: 8g, Fiber: 6g

Black Bean and Corn Quesadillas

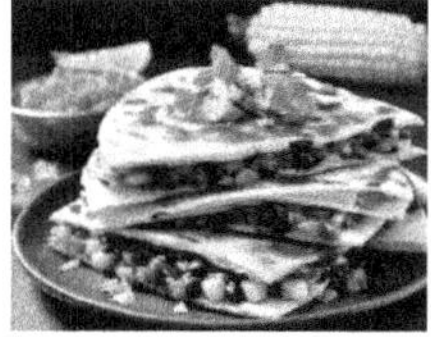

These gluten-free quesadillas are filled with a savory mixture of black beans, corn, and spices, making them a satisfying and flavorful lunch option.
Preparation Time: 10 minutes
Cooking Time: 10 minutes
Total Time: 20 minutes
Servings: 2
Ingredients
4 gluten-free tortillas
1 can black beans, drained and rinsed
1 cup corn kernels
1/2 cup diced red bell pepper
1/4 cup chopped fresh cilantro
1 teaspoon ground cumin
1/2 teaspoon chili powder
Salt and pepper to taste
1 cup shredded vegan cheese
Guacamole and salsa for serving
Instructions
1. In a large bowl, combine black beans, corn kernels, diced red bell pepper, chopped fresh cilantro, ground cumin, chili powder, salt, and pepper.
2. Place a gluten-free tortilla on a flat surface.
3. Spread a quarter of the black bean mixture evenly over half of the tortilla.
4. Sprinkle a quarter of the shredded vegan cheese over the black bean mixture.
5. Fold the tortilla in half to cover the filling.
6. Repeat the process with the remaining tortillas and filling.
7. Heat a large skillet over medium-high heat.
8. Place the quesadillas in the skillet and cook for 3-4 minutes on each side, until golden brown and crispy.
9. Cut each quesadilla into wedges and serve with guacamole and salsa.
Nutritional Info: Calories: 320, Protein: 12g, Carbohydrates: 40g, Fat: 14g, Fiber: 8g

Millet Salad with grapefruit and orange

A refreshing salad bursting with citrus flavors and hearty millet.
Preparation Time: 15 minutes
Cooking Time: 20 minutes
Total Time: 35 minutes
Servings: 2
Ingredients
1 cup cooked millet
1 orange, segmented
1 grapefruit, segmented
1 carrot, grated
2 tablespoons chopped almonds
2 tablespoons chopped fresh parsley
Salt and pepper to taste
Instructions

1. In a bowl, combine cooked millet, orange segments, grapefruit segments, grated carrot, chopped almonds, and parsley.
2. Season the salad with salt and pepper to taste.
3. Toss gently to combine.
4. Serve chilled.
Nutritional Info: Calories: 220, Protein: 6g, Carbohydrates: 40g, Fat: 5g, Fiber: 7g

Almond-Crusted Tofu with Citrus Glaze

Crispy almond-crusted tofu served with a tangy citrus glaze.
Preparation Time: 15 minutes
Cooking Time: 20 minutes
Total Time: 35 minutes
Servings: 2
Ingredients
1 block tofu, pressed and sliced into cubes
1/4 cup almond flour
1 teaspoon garlic powder
1 teaspoon smoked paprika
Salt and pepper to taste
Zest of 1 orange
Juice of 1 orange
Juice of 1 lemon
2 tablespoons maple syrup
Instructions
1. Preheat oven to 375°F (190°C). Line a baking sheet with parchment paper.
2. In a bowl, mix almond flour, garlic powder, smoked paprika, salt, pepper, and orange zest.
3. Coat tofu cubes with the almond flour mixture and place them on the prepared baking sheet.
4. Bake for 15-20 minutes or until tofu is crispy and golden.
5. In a small saucepan, combine orange juice, lemon juice, and maple syrup.
6. Simmer until slightly thickened.
7. Drizzle the citrus glaze over the baked tofu before serving.
Nutritional Info: Calories: 320, Protein: 18g, Carbohydrates: 25g, Fat: 15g, Fiber: 5g

Carrot and Apple Soup

A comforting soup made with carrots, apples, and warming spices.
Preparation Time: 10 minutes
Cooking Time: 25 minutes
Total Time: 35 minutes
Servings: 4
Ingredients
4 large carrots, peeled and chopped
2 apples, peeled, cored, and chopped
1 onion, chopped
3 cups vegetable broth

1 teaspoon ground cumin
1/2 teaspoon ground cinnamon
Salt and pepper to taste
2 tablespoons olive oil
Chopped fresh parsley for garnish
Instructions
1. In a large pot, heat the oil over medium-high heat.
2. Add the onion and sauté until translucent.
3. Add chopped carrots and apples to the pot.
4. Cook for 5 minutes, stirring occasionally.
5. Stir in ground cumin, ground cinnamon, salt, and pepper.
6. Pour in vegetable broth and bring to a boil.
7. Reduce heat and simmer for 15-20 minutes, or until carrots and apples are tender.
8. Remove from heat and let cool slightly and then, use an immersion blender to blend the soup until smooth.
9. Serve hot, garnished with chopped fresh parsley.
Nutritional Info: Calories: 180, Protein: 2g, Carbohydrates: 25g, Fat: 9g, Fiber: 5g

Apple and Almond Butter Sandwich

A simple yet satisfying sandwich featuring crisp apple slices and creamy almond butter.
Preparation Time: 5 minutes
Total Time: 5 minutes
Serving: 1
Ingredients
2 slices gluten-free bread
2 tablespoons almond butter
1 apple, thinly sliced
Cinnamon for sprinkling (optional)
Instructions
1. Spread almond butter evenly on one slice of bread.
2. Arrange apple slices on top of the almond butter.
3. Sprinkle with cinnamon if desired.
4. Top with the second slice of bread.
5. Cut in half and serve.
Nutritional Info: Calories: 320, Protein: 8g, Carbohydrates: 45g, Fat: 14g, Fiber: 9g

Quinoa Salad with Almonds

A light and zesty salad featuring fluffy quinoa, citrus fruits, and crunchy almonds.
Preparation Time: 10 minutes
Cooking Time: 20 minutes
Total Time: 30 minutes
Servings: 2
Ingredients
1 cup cooked quinoa
1 orange, segmented

1 grapefruit, segmented
1/4 cup sliced almonds
2 tablespoons chopped fresh mint
2 tablespoons olive oil
1 tablespoon lemon juice
Salt and pepper to taste
Instructions
1. In a bowl, combine cooked quinoa, orange segments, grapefruit segments, sliced almonds, and chopped fresh mint.
2. In a small jar, whisk together olive oil, lemon juice, salt, and pepper to make the dressing.
3. Pour the dressing over the quinoa salad and toss gently to combine.
4. Serve chilled or at room temperature.
Nutritional Info: Calories: 280, Protein: 7g, Carbohydrates: 35g, Fat: 12g, Fiber: 6g

Carrot and Millet Patties

Delicious patties made with shredded carrots, cooked millet, and aromatic spices.
Preparation Time: 15 minutes
Cooking Time: 20 minutes
Total Time: 35 minutes
Servings: 4
Ingredients
1 cup cooked millet
1 cup shredded carrots
1/4 cup almond flour
2 tablespoons chopped fresh cilantro
1 teaspoon ground cumin
1/2 teaspoon ground coriander
Salt and pepper to taste
Olive oil for frying
Instructions
1. In a large bowl, combine cooked millet, shredded carrots, almond flour, chopped fresh cilantro, ground cumin, ground coriander, salt, and pepper.
2. Mix until well combined.
3. Shape the mixture into patties.
4. Heat the oil in a skillet over medium-high heat.
5. Fry the patties for 3-4 minutes on each side or until golden brown and crispy.
6. Serve hot with your favorite dipping sauce or in a salad.
Nutritional Info: Calories: 200, Protein: 5g, Carbohydrates: 30g, Fat: 7g, Fiber: 5g

Almond Flour Crusted Citrus Tilapia

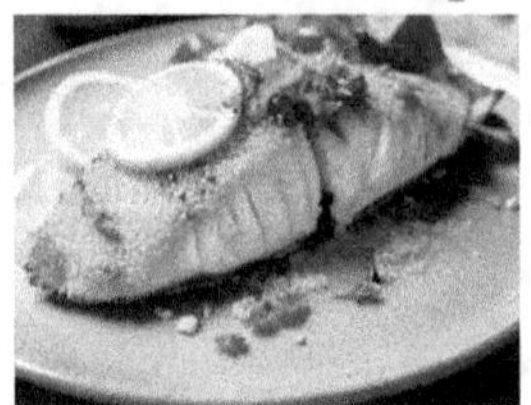

Tilapia fillets coated in almond flour and citrus zest, then baked to perfection.
Preparation Time: 10 minutes
Cooking Time: 15 minutes
Total Time: 25 minutes
Servings: 2
Ingredients
2 tilapia fillets
1/4 cup almond flour
Zest of 1 lemon
Zest of 1 orange
Salt and pepper to taste
Olive oil spray
Instructions
1. Preheat oven to 400°F (200°C).
2. Line a baking sheet with parchment paper and lightly grease with olive oil spray.
3. In a shallow dish, combine almond flour, lemon zest, orange zest, salt, and pepper.
4. Pat tilapia fillets dry with paper towels, then dredge them in the almond flour mixture, pressing gently to adhere.
5. Place the coated fillets on the prepared baking sheet.
6. Lightly spray the tops of the fillets with olive oil spray.
7. Bake for 12-15 minutes or until fish is cooked through and crust is golden brown.
8. Serve hot with a squeeze of fresh lemon or orange juice.
Nutritional Info: Calories: 280, Protein: 30g, Carbohydrates: 5g, Fat: 15g, Fiber: 2g

Apple and Carrot Coleslaw

A refreshing coleslaw with crisp apples, shredded carrots, and a tangy dressing.
Preparation Time: 10 minutes
Total Time: 10 minutes
Servings: 4
Ingredients
2 apples, julienned
2 carrots, grated
1/4 cup sliced almonds
1/4 cup dairy-free yogurt
2 tablespoons lemon juice
1 tablespoon maple syrup

Salt and pepper to taste

Instructions

1. In a large bowl, combine julienned apples, grated carrots, and sliced almonds.
2. In a small bowl, whisk together dairy-free yogurt, lemon juice, maple syrup, salt, and pepper to make the dressing.
3. Pour the dressing over the apple and carrot mixture.
4. Toss gently to coat everything evenly.
5. Serve chilled.

Nutritional Info: Calories: 180, Protein: 3g, Carbohydrates: 25g, Fat: 8g, Fiber: 6g

Almond Energy Balls with orange and lemon

Nutrient-packed energy balls with a burst of citrus flavor and crunchy almonds.

Preparation Time: 10 minutes

Total Time: 10 minutes

Servings: Makes 12 balls

Ingredients

1 cup almond flour

1/2 cup shredded coconut

Zest of 1 lemon

Zest of 1 orange

1/4 cup almond butter

2 tablespoons maple syrup

1 tablespoon lemon juice

1/4 cup chopped almonds

Instructions

1. In a large bowl, mix together almond flour, shredded coconut, lemon zest, and orange zest.
2. Add almond butter, maple syrup, and lemon juice to the dry ingredients. Stir until well combined.
3. Fold in chopped almonds.
4. Use your hands to roll the mixture into small balls.
5. Transfer to a baking sheet lined with parchment paper.
6. Place in a fridge for at least 30 minutes to firm up.
7. Serve chilled as a snack or dessert.

Nutritional Info: Calories: 120, Protein: 3g, Carbohydrates: 10g, Fat: 8g, Fiber: 2g

Buckwheat Salad with Carrots and Almonds

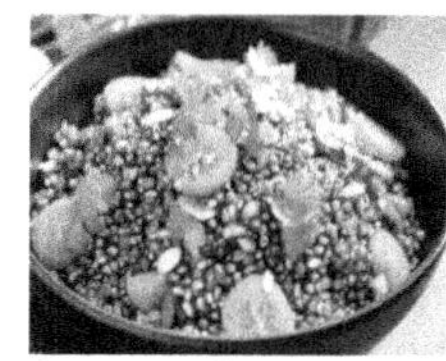

A refreshing salad with nutty buckwheat, crunchy carrots, and zesty citrus flavors.

Preparation Time: 15 minutes

Cooking Time: 15 minutes

Total Time: 30 minutes
Servings: 2
Ingredients
1 cup cooked buckwheat groats
1 large carrot, grated
1 orange, segmented
1/4 cup sliced almonds
2 tablespoons chopped fresh parsley
Zest of 1 lemon
Juice of 1 lemon
2 tablespoons olive oil
Salt and pepper to taste
Instructions
1. In a large bowl, combine cooked buckwheat groats, grated carrot, orange segments, sliced almonds, and chopped parsley.
2. In a small jar, whisk together lemon zest, lemon juice, olive oil, salt, and pepper to make the dressing.
3. Pour the dressing over the salad and toss gently until just coated.
4. Serve chilled or at room temperature.
Nutritional Info: Calories: 320, Protein: 8g, Carbohydrates: 45g, Fat: 14g, Fiber: 8g

Carrot and Citrus Buckwheat Wraps

Vibrant wraps filled with shredded carrots, citrusy buckwheat, and crunchy seeds.
Preparation Time: 20 minutes
Cooking Time: 15 minutes
Total Time: 35 minutes
Servings: 4
Ingredients
1 cup cooked buckwheat groats
2 large carrots, shredded
Zest of 1 orange
Juice of 1 orange
Zest of 1 lemon
Juice of 1 lemon
1 tablespoon olive oil
1 tablespoon maple syrup
1/4 cup mixed seeds (such as sunflower seeds, pumpkin seeds, and sesame seeds)
4 gluten-free wraps
Instructions
1. In a large bowl, combine cooked buckwheat groats, shredded carrots, orange zest, lemon zest, orange juice, lemon juice, olive oil, and maple syrup.
2. Mix in mixed seeds.
3. Divide the buckwheat mixture evenly among the gluten-free wraps.
4. Roll up the wraps tightly.
5. Slice in half and serve.
Nutritional Info: Calories: 280, Protein: 6g, Carbohydrates: 35g, Fat: 12g, Fiber: 7g

Roasted Carrot and Chickpea Salad with Quinoa

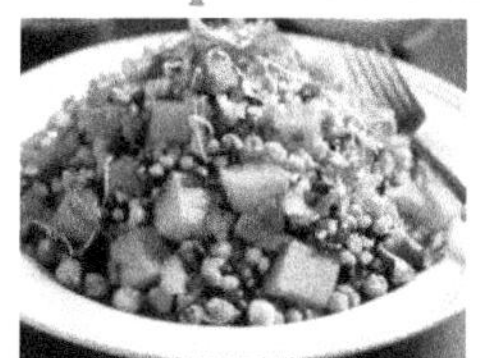

A hearty salad with roasted carrots, protein-rich chickpeas, fluffy quinoa, and citrus dressing.
Preparation Time: 15 minutes
Cooking Time: 30 minutes
Total Time: 45 minutes
Servings: 4
Ingredients
1 cup quinoa, rinsed
4 large carrots, peeled and sliced into sticks
1 can (15 oz.) chickpeas, drained and rinsed
Zest of 1 orange
Juice of 1 orange
Zest of 1 lemon
Juice of 1 lemon
2 tablespoons olive oil
Salt and pepper to taste
Fresh parsley for garnish
Instructions
1. Preheat oven to 400°F (200°C).
2. In a large bowl, toss carrot sticks with olive oil, orange zest, lemon zest, salt, and pepper.
3. Spread carrots on a baking sheet and roast for 25-30 minutes, or until tender and caramelized.
4. Meanwhile, cook quinoa following the package instructions.
5. In a small bowl, whisk together orange juice, lemon juice, and a drizzle of olive oil to make the dressing.
6. In a large bowl, combine cooked quinoa, roasted carrots, chickpeas, and dressing. Toss to combine.
7. Garnish with fresh parsley before serving.
Nutritional Info: Calories: 320, Protein: 10g, Carbohydrates: 50g, Fat: 8g, Fiber: 10g

Buckwheat and Carrot Soup with Citrus Twist

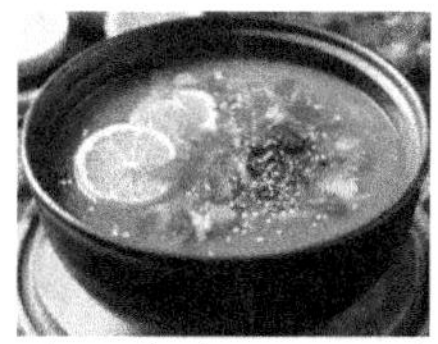

A comforting soup made with earthy buckwheat, sweet carrots, and a burst of citrus flavor.

Preparation Time: 10 minutes
Cooking Time: 25 minutes
Total Time: 35 minutes
Serving Size: 4

Ingredients

1 cup raw buckwheat groats
4 large carrots, peeled and chopped
1 onion, chopped
Zest of 1 orange
Juice of 1 orange
Zest of 1 lemon
Juice of 1 lemon
4 cups vegetable broth
Salt and pepper to taste
2 tablespoons olive oil

Instructions

1. In a large pot, heat the oil over medium-high heat. Add chopped onion and sauté until translucent.
2. Add chopped carrots and raw buckwheat groats to the pot. Cook for 5 minutes, stirring occasionally.
3. Pour in vegetable broth, orange zest, lemon zest, orange juice, and lemon juice. Bring to a boil.
4. Reduce heat and simmer for 15-20 minutes, or until buckwheat and carrots are tender.
5. Blend the soup with an immersion blender until smooth.
6. Season the soup with salt and pepper to taste.
7. Serve hot, garnished with a slice of orange if desired.

Nutritional Info: Calories: 280, Protein: 8g, Carbohydrates: 45g, Fat: 10g, Fiber: 8g

Assorted Seeds Salad

A vibrant salad featuring shredded carrots, assorted seeds, and a tangy citrus dressing.

Preparation Time: 10 minutes
Total Time: 10 minutes
Servings: 2

Ingredients

2 cups shredded carrots
2 tablespoons sunflower seeds
2 tablespoons pumpkin seeds
2 tablespoons sesame seeds
Zest of 1 orange
Zest of 1 lemon
Juice of 1 orange
Juice of 1 lemon
1 tablespoon olive oil
1 teaspoon honey or maple syrup (optional)
Salt and pepper to taste

Instructions
1. In a large bowl, combine shredded carrots, sunflower seeds, pumpkin seeds, sesame seeds, orange zest, and lemon zest.
2. In a small jar, whisk together orange juice, lemon juice, olive oil, honey or maple syrup (if using), salt, and pepper to make the dressing.
3. Pour the dressing on the salad and toss gently to combine.
4. Serve chilled or at room temperature.
Nutritional Info: Calories: 220, Protein: 6g, Carbohydrates: 30g, Fat: 10g, Fiber: 8g

Buckwheat Stir-Fry with Tofu and Carrots

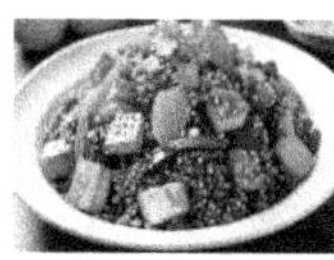

A flavorful stir-fry featuring buckwheat, tofu, carrots, and a zesty citrus sauce.
Preparation Time: 20 minutes
Cooking Time: 15 minutes
Total Time: 35 minutes
Servings: 4
Ingredients
1 cup raw buckwheat groats
1 block tofu, pressed and cubed
2 large carrots, julienned
1 bell pepper, sliced
Zest of 1 orange
Zest of 1 lemon
Juice of 1 orange
Juice of 1 lemon
2 tablespoons soy sauce or tamari
1 tablespoon maple syrup
2 cloves garlic, minced
1 tablespoon grated ginger
2 tablespoons sesame oil
Salt and pepper to taste
Sesame seeds for garnish
Instructions
1. Cook buckwheat groats according to package instructions. Set aside.
2. In a small bowl, whisk together orange zest, lemon zest, orange juice, lemon juice, soy sauce or tamari, maple syrup, garlic, and ginger to make the sauce.
3. Heat sesame oil in a large skillet or wok over medium-high heat.
4. Add tofu cubes and cook until golden brown on all sides. Remove from the skillet and set aside.
5. In the same skillet, add julienned carrots and sliced bell pepper. Stir-fry until vegetables are tender-crisp, for about 4 minutes..

6. Add cooked buckwheat, tofu, and the prepared sauce to the skillet. Stir-fry for another 2-3 minutes, or until everything is heated through and well coated in the sauce.
7. Season with salt and pepper to taste.
8. Serve hot, garnished with sesame seeds.
Nutritional Info: Calories: 350, Protein: 15g, Carbohydrates: 45g, Fat: 12g, Fiber: 8g

Carrot and Citrus Buckwheat Bowl

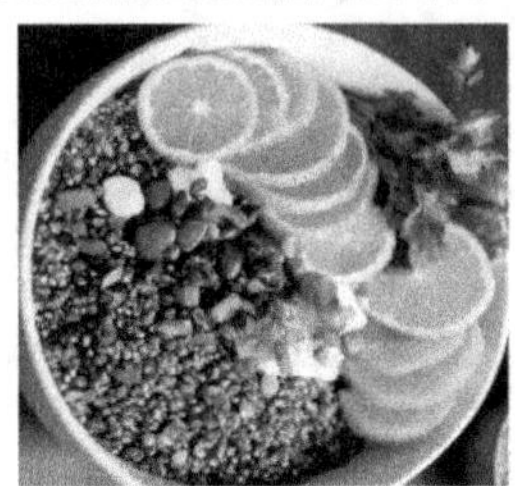

A nourishing bowl featuring cooked buckwheat, shredded carrots, and fresh citrus segments.
Preparation Time: 10 minutes
Cooking Time: 15 minutes
Total Time: 25 minutes
Servings: 2
Ingredients
1 cup cooked buckwheat groats
1 large carrot, shredded
1 orange, segmented
1/4 cup sliced almonds
2 tablespoons hemp seeds
Zest of 1 lemon
Juice of 1 lemon
2 tablespoons olive oil
Salt and pepper to taste
Instructions
1. In a large bowl, combine cooked buckwheat groats, shredded carrot, orange segments, sliced almonds, hemp seeds, and lemon zest.
2. In a small jar, whisk together lemon juice, olive oil, salt, and pepper to make the dressing.
3. Pour the dressing over the buckwheat bowl and toss gently to combine.
4. Serve warm or at room temperature.
Nutritional Info: Calories: 320, Protein: 10g, Carbohydrates: 40g, Fat: 15g, Fiber: 8g

Nutrient-packed energy balls

This Nutrient-packed energy balls with shredded carrots, citrus zest, and an assortment of seeds.
Preparation Time: 15 minutes
Total Time: 15 minutes
Servings: Makes 12 balls
Ingredients

1 cup shredded carrots
1 cup rolled oats (gluten-free)
1/2 cup almond butter
1/4 cup maple syrup
Zest of 1 orange
Zest of 1 lemon
1/4 cup mixed seeds (such as pumpkin seeds, sunflower seeds, and chia seeds)
Pinch of salt

Instructions

1. In a food processor, combine shredded carrots, rolled oats, almond butter, maple syrup, orange zest, lemon zest, mixed seeds, and a pinch of salt.
2. Pulse until the mixture forms a sticky dough.
3. Scoop out tablespoon-sized portions of the dough and roll into balls using your hands.
4. Place the energy balls on a baking sheet lined with parchment paper.
5. Refrigerate for at least 30 minutes to firm up.
6. Serve chilled as a snack or dessert.

Nutritional Info: Calories: 180, Protein: 5g, Carbohydrates: 20g, Fat: 9g, Fiber: 4g

DINNER

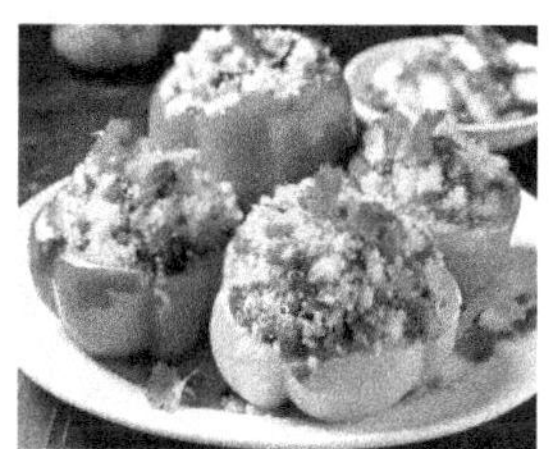

Quinoa Stuffed Bell Peppers

Colorful bell peppers stuffed with protein-rich quinoa, black beans, corn, and spices.

Preparation Time: 15 minutes
Cooking Time: 30 minutes
Total Time: 45 minutes
Servings: 4

Ingredients

4 large bell peppers
1 cup cooked quinoa
1 can (15 oz.) black beans, drained and rinsed
1 cup corn kernels (fresh or frozen)
1 small onion, diced
2 cloves garlic, minced
1 teaspoon ground cumin
1/2 teaspoon chili powder

Salt and pepper to taste
1/4 cup chopped fresh cilantro
1 cup tomato sauce
Optional toppings: avocado, vegan cheese
Instruction
1. Preheat the oven to 375°F (190°C). Grease a baking dish.
2. Cut the tops off the bell peppers and remove the seeds and membranes.
3. In a large bowl, mix together cooked quinoa, black beans, corn, onion, garlic, cumin, chili powder, salt, pepper, and cilantro.
4. Stuff each bell pepper with the quinoa mixture and place them in the prepared baking dish.
5. Pour tomato sauce over the stuffed peppers.
6. Cover the dish with foil and bake for 25-30 minutes, or until the peppers are tender.
7. Serve hot, topped with avocado slices and vegan cheese if desired.
Nutritional Info: Calories: 300, Protein: 12g, Carbohydrates: 45g, Fat: 8g, Fiber: 10g

Coconut Curry with Tofu and Vegetables

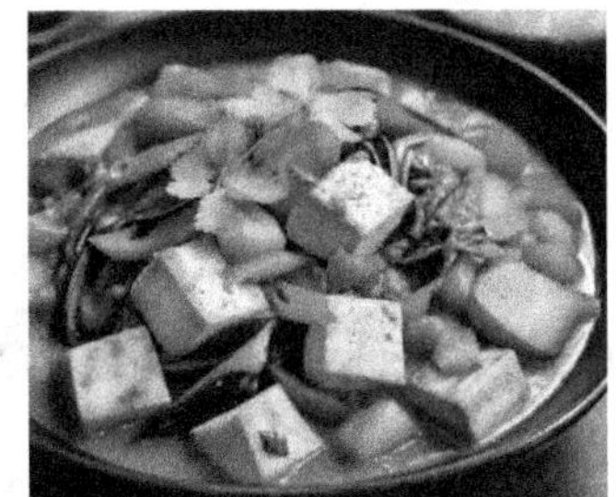

Creamy coconut curry loaded with tofu, bell peppers, broccoli, and aromatic spices.
Preparation Time: 20 minutes
Cooking Time: 25 minutes
Total Time: 45 minutes
Servings: 4
Ingredients
1 block firm tofu, pressed and cubed
2 tablespoons coconut oil
1 onion, diced
3 cloves garlic, minced
1 tablespoon grated ginger
1 red bell pepper, sliced
1 yellow bell pepper, sliced
1 cup broccoli florets
2 tablespoons curry powder
1 can (14 oz) coconut milk
1 tablespoon soy sauce or tamari
Juice of 1 lime
Salt and pepper to taste

F resh cilantro for garnish

Instructions

1. Heat the oil in a large skillet over medium heat.

2. Add cubed tofu and cook until golden brown on all sides.

3. Remove tofu from the skillet and set aside.

4. In the same skillet, add diced onion, minced garlic, and grated ginger. Cook until fragrant.

Vegetable Stir-Fry with Tamari Glaze

Quick and easy vegetable stir-fry with a savory tamari glaze, served over gluten-free rice or noodles.

Preparation Time: 15 minutes

Cooking Time: 15 minutes

Total Time: 30 minutes

Servings: 4

Ingredients

2 tablespoons sesame oil

2 cloves garlic, minced

1 tablespoon grated ginger

2 cups mixed vegetables (such as bell peppers, broccoli, snap peas, carrots)

1/4 cup tamari or soy sauce

2 tablespoons maple syrup

1 tablespoon rice vinegar

1 tablespoon cornstarch mixed with 2 tablespoons water

Cooked rice or gluten-free noodles for serving

Sesame seeds and green onions for garnish

Instructions

1. Heat sesame oil in a large skillet or wok over medium-high heat.

2. Add minced garlic and grated ginger. Cook until fragrant.

3. Add mixed vegetables to the skillet and stir-fry until tender-crisp.

4. In a small bowl, whisk together tamari or soy sauce, maple syrup, rice vinegar, and cornstarch mixture.

5. Pour the sauce over the vegetables in the skillet and cook, stirring constantly, until the sauce thickens and coats the vegetables.

7. Serve hot over cooked rice or gluten-free noodles.

8. Garnish with sesame seeds and sliced green onions and enjoy.

Nutritional Info: Calories: 250, Protein: 5g, Carbohydrates: 35g, Fat: 10g, Fiber: 6g

Spaghetti Squash Pad Thai

A gluten-free twist on the classic Pad Thai using spaghetti squash instead of noodles, topped with tofu and vegetables.

Preparation Time: 15 minutes

Cooking Time: 45 minutes

Total Time: 1 hour

Servings: 4

Ingredients

1 large spaghetti squash

1 block firm tofu, pressed and cubed

2 tablespoons sesame oil
2 cloves garlic, minced
1 tablespoon grated ginger
2 cups mixed vegetables (such as bell peppers, bean sprouts, carrots, green onions)
1/4 cup tamari or soy sauce
2 tablespoons maple syrup
Juice of 1 lime
Crushed peanuts and fresh cilantro for garnish

Instructions

1. Preheat the oven to 400°F (200°C). Cut the spaghetti squash in half lengthwise, make sure you scoop out the seeds.
2. Place the squash halves cut-side down on a baking sheet.
3. Roast in the oven for 35-45 minutes, or until tender and easily pierced with a fork. Let cool slightly.
4. While the squash is roasting, heat sesame oil in a large skillet over medium heat.
5. Add minced garlic and grated ginger. Cook until fragrant.
6. Add cubed tofu to the skillet and cook until golden brown on all sides.
7. Add mixed vegetables to the skillet and stir-fry until tender-crisp.
8. In a small bowl, whisk together tamari or soy sauce, maple syrup, and lime juice.
9. Use a fork to scrape the spaghetti squash strands into the skillet with the tofu and vegetables.
10. Pour the sauce over the squash mixture and toss to combine.
11. Serve hot, garnished with crushed peanuts and fresh cilantro.

Nutritional Info: Calories: 280, Protein: 10g, Carbohydrates: 35g, Fat: 12g, Fiber: 8g

Mushroom and Spinach Risotto

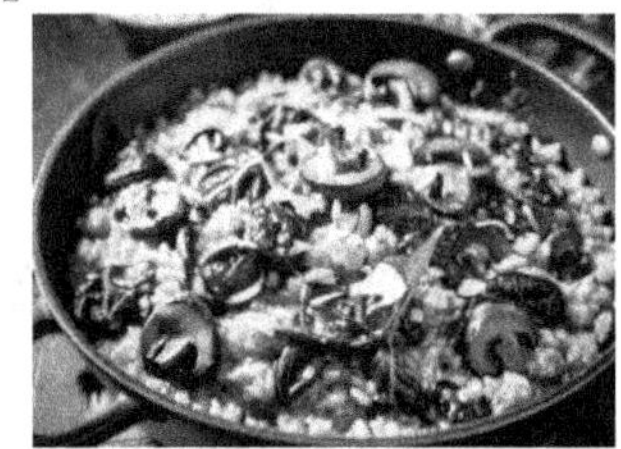

Creamy risotto made with Arborio rice, mushrooms, spinach, and vegetable broth.

Preparation Time: 10 minutes
Cooking Time: 30 minutes
Total Time: 40 minutes
Servings: 4

Ingredients

1 tablespoon olive oil
1 onion, diced
2 cloves garlic, minced
8 oz mushrooms, sliced
1 cup Arborio rice
4 cups vegetable broth, warmed
2 cups baby spinach

1/4 cup nutritional yeast (optional)
Salt and pepper to taste
Fresh parsley for garnish

Instructions

1. Heat olive oil in a large pot or skillet over medium-high heat.
2. Add diced onion and minced garlic. Cook until softened.
3. Add sliced mushrooms to the skillet and cook until browned and tender.
4. Stir in Arborio rice and cook for 1-2 minutes until lightly toasted.
5. Begin adding warmed vegetable broth to the skillet, 1 cup at a time, stirring frequently and allowing the liquid to absorb before adding more.
6. Continue cooking and stirring until the rice is creamy and cooked through, about 20-25 minutes.
7. Stir in baby spinach and nutritional yeast, if using. Cook until spinach is wilted.
8. Season the mushroom and spinach risotto with salt and pepper to taste.
9. Serve hot, garnished with fresh parsley.

Nutritional Info: Calories: 300, Protein: 8g, Carbohydrates: 50g, Fat: 6g, Fiber: 6g

Eggplant Involtini with Vegan Ricotta

Thinly sliced eggplant filled with creamy vegan ricotta cheese, rolled up and baked with marinara sauce.

Preparation Time: 20 minutes
Cooking Time: 40 minutes
Total Time: 1 hour
Servings: 4

Ingredients

2 large eggplants, sliced lengthwise into thin strips
1 tablespoon olive oil
1 cup vegan ricotta cheese
1/4 cup nutritional yeast
2 tablespoons chopped fresh basil
Salt and pepper to taste
2 cups marinara sauce
Vegan Parmesan cheese for topping

Instructions

1. Preheat the oven to 375°F (190°C). Grease a baking dish with olive oil.
2. Place eggplant slices on a baking sheet and brush both sides with olive oil.
3. Bake for 10-12 minutes, or until softened.
4. In a bowl, mix together vegan ricotta cheese, nutritional yeast, chopped fresh basil, salt, and pepper.
5. Spread one spoonful of marinara sauce on each eggplant slice and place a dollop of vegan ricotta mixture at one end of each slice and roll up.
6. Place the rolled eggplant slices seam-side down in the prepared baking dish.
7. Pour remaining marinara sauce over the top of the eggplant rolls.
8. Bake for 25-30 minutes, or until heated through and bubbly.
9. Serve hot, sprinkled with vegan Parmesan cheese.

Nutritional Info: Calories: 280, Protein: 10g, Carbohydrates: 30g, Fat: 12g, Fiber: 8g

Chickpea and Vegetable Curry

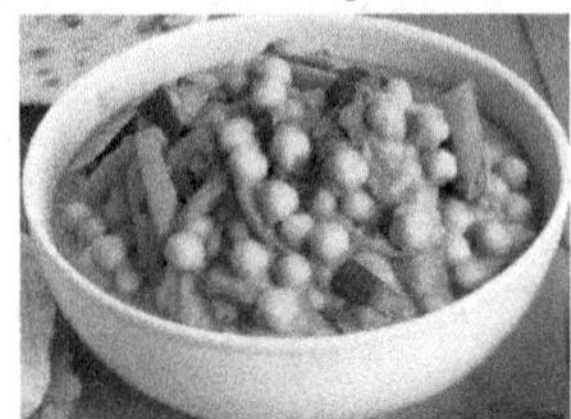

Flavorful curry made with chickpeas, mixed vegetables, and aromatic spices, served over rice or quinoa.
Preparation Time: 15 minutes
Cooking Time: 25 minutes
Total Time: 40 minutes
Servings: 4
Ingredients
1 tablespoon coconut oil
1 onion, diced
3 cloves garlic, minced
1 tablespoon grated ginger
2 tablespoons curry powder
1 can (15 oz.) chickpeas, drained and rinsed
2 cups mixed vegetables (such as bell peppers, cauliflower, peas, carrots)
1 can (14 oz.) coconut milk
1 cup vegetable broth
Salt and pepper to taste
Cooked rice or quinoa for serving
Fresh cilantro for garnish
Instructions
1. Heat coconut oil in a large skillet or pot over medium heat.
2. Add diced onion, minced garlic, and grated ginger. Cook until softened.
3. Stir in curry powder and cook for one more minute until fragrant.
4. Add chickpeas, mixed vegetables, coconut milk, and vegetable broth to the skillet. Bring to a simmer.
5. Simmer for 15-20 minutes, or until vegetables are tender and the curry has thickened.
6. Season with salt and pepper to taste.
7. Serve hot over cooked rice or quinoa, garnished with fresh cilantro.
Nutritional Info: Calories: 320, Protein: 10g, Carbohydrates: 40g, Fat: 15g, Fiber: 10g

Stuffed Portobello Mushrooms

Large portobello mushrooms filled with a savory mixture of quinoa, vegetables, and vegan cheese.
Preparation Time: 15 minutes
Cooking Time: 25 minutes
Total Time: 40 minutes
Servings: 4
Ingredients

4 large portobello mushrooms, stems removed
1 tablespoon olive oil
1 onion, diced
2 cloves garlic, minced
1 bell pepper, diced
1 cup cooked quinoa
1/2 cup marinara sauce
1/2 cup vegan cheese shreds
Salt and pepper to taste
Fresh parsley for garnish

Instructions

1. Preheat the oven to 375°F (190°C). Grease a baking sheet.
2. Place portobello mushrooms on the baking sheet, gill-side up.
3. In a skillet, heat oil over medium-high heat.
4. Add diced onion, minced garlic, and diced bell pepper. Cook until softened.
5. Stir in cooked quinoa and marinara sauce. Cook for another 2-3 minutes.
6. Spoon the quinoa mixture into the portobello mushroom caps.
7. Top each stuffed mushroom with vegan cheese shreds.
8. Bake for 20-25 minutes, or until mushrooms are tender and cheese is melted and bubbly.
9. Serve hot, garnished with fresh parsley.

Nutritional Info: Calories: 250, Protein: 8g, Carbohydrates: 30g, Fat: 10g, Fiber: 6g

Sweet Potato and Black Bean Enchiladas

Flavorful enchiladas filled with mashed sweet potatoes, black beans, and spices, topped with enchilada sauce.

Preparation Time: 20 minutes
Cooking Time: 30 minutes
Total Time: 50 minutes
Servings: 4

Ingredients

2 large sweet potatoes, peeled and diced
1 can (15 oz) black beans, drained and rinsed
1 onion, diced
2 cloves garlic, minced
1 teaspoon ground cumin
1/2 teaspoon chili powder
Salt and pepper to taste
8 gluten-free tortillas
2 cups enchilada sauce
Vegan cheese shreds for topping
Fresh cilantro for garnish

Instructions

1. Preheat the oven to 375°F (190°C). Grease a baking dish.
2. Place diced sweet potatoes in a pot of boiling water.
3. Cook until tender, about 10-15 minutes. Drain and mash with a fork.

4. In a skillet, heat the oil over medium heat. Add diced onion and minced garlic. Cook until softened.
5. Stir in mashed sweet potatoes, black beans, ground cumin, chili powder, salt, and pepper. Cook for another 2-3 minutes.
6. Spoon the sweet potato and black bean mixture onto each tortilla, roll up, and place seam-side down in the prepared baking dish.
7. Pour enchilada sauce over the top of the rolled tortillas.
8. Sprinkle vegan cheese shreds over the enchiladas.
9. Bake for 20-25 minutes, or until heated through and bubbly.
10. Serve hot, garnished with fresh cilantro.
Nutritional Info: Calories: 300, Protein: 10g, Carbohydrates: 40g, Fat: 12g, Fiber: 8g

Lentil and Vegetable Curry

Hearty curry made with lentils, vegetables, and aromatic spices, served over rice.
Preparation Time: 10 minutes
Cooking Time: 30 minutes
Total Time: 40 minutes
Servings: 4
Ingredients
1 cup dried lentils, rinsed
2 cups vegetable broth
1 onion, diced
2 cloves garlic, minced
1 tablespoon curry powder
1 teaspoon turmeric
1 teaspoon cumin
1 can (14 oz) coconut milk
2 cups chopped mixed vegetables (e.g., carrots, cauliflower, bell peppers)
Salt and pepper to taste
Cooked rice for serving
Instructions
1. In a large pot, combine lentils, vegetable broth, onion, garlic, curry powder, turmeric, and cumin.
2. Bring to a boil, then reduce heat and simmer for 20 minutes or until lentils are tender.
3. Stir in coconut milk and mixed vegetables.
4. Simmer for an additional 10 minutes until vegetables are cooked through.
5. Season with salt and pepper.
6. Serve over cooked rice.
Nutritional Info: Calories: 380, Protein: 15g, Carbohydrates: 50g, Fat: 15g, Fiber: 12g

Chickpea and Vegetable Stir-Fry

Quick and easy stir-fry loaded with chickpeas, colorful vegetables, and a savory sauce.
Preparation Time: 10 minutes
Cooking Time: 15 minutes
Total Time: 25 minutes

Servings: 2
Ingredients
1 can (15 oz.) chickpeas, drained and rinsed
2 cups mixed vegetables (such as bell peppers, broccoli, snap peas)
1 onion, sliced
2 cloves garlic, minced
2 tablespoons soy sauce or tamari
1 tablespoon maple syrup
1 tablespoon sesame oil
Cooked rice or quinoa for serving
Instructions
1. Heat sesame oil in a large skillet over medium heat.
2. Add onion and garlic, sauté until fragrant.
3. Add mixed vegetables and chickpeas, stir-fry for 5-7 minutes until vegetables are tender.
4. In a small bowl, whisk together soy sauce and maple syrup.
5. Pour the sauce over the stir-fry and toss to coat.
6. Cook for another 2-3 minutes.
7. Serve hot over cooked rice or quinoa.
Nutritional Info: Calories: 380, Protein: 12g, Carbohydrates: 55g, Fat: 10g, Fiber: 10g

Mediterranean Quinoa Salad

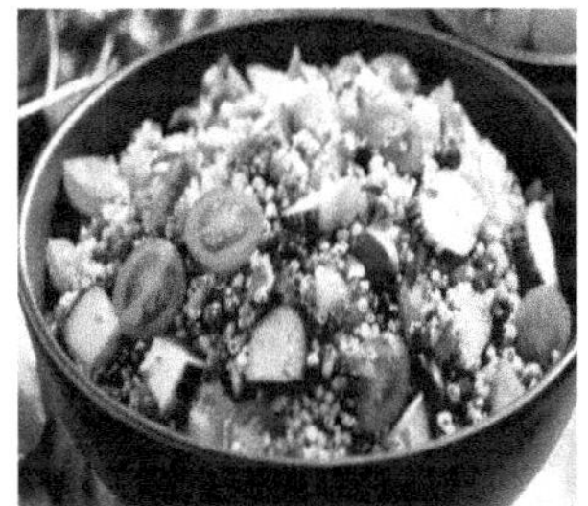

Refreshing salad with quinoa, fresh vegetables, olives, and a zesty lemon dressing.
Preparation Time: 15 minutes
Cooking Time: 15 minutes (for quinoa)
Total Time: 30 minutes
Servings: 4
Ingredients
1 cup cooked quinoa
1 cucumber, diced
1 cup cherry tomatoes, halved
1/2 cup sliced Kalamata olives
1/4 cup chopped fresh parsley
1/4 cup diced red onion
Juice of 1 lemon
2 tablespoons olive oil
Salt and pepper to taste
Instructions

1. In a large bowl, combine cooked quinoa, cucumber, cherry tomatoes, olives, parsley, and red onion.
2. In a small bowl, whisk together lemon juice, olive oil, salt, and pepper to make the dressing.
3. Pour the dressing on the salad and toss to combine.
4. Serve chilled or at room temperature.
Nutritional Info: Calories: 280, Protein: 6g, Carbohydrates: 35g, Fat: 12g, Fiber: 6g

Butternut Squash and Chickpea Buddha Bowl

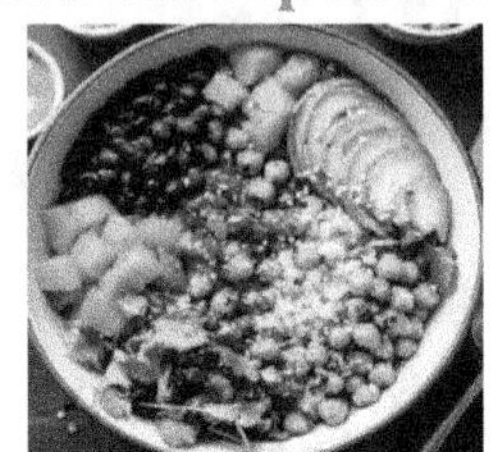

Nourishing Buddha bowl featuring roasted butternut squash, chickpeas, and a variety of colorful vegetables.

Preparation Time: 15 minutes
Cooking Time: 25 minutes
Total Time: 40 minutes
Servings: 2

Ingredients

2 cups cubed butternut squash
1 can (15 oz.) chickpeas, drained and rinsed
2 cups mixed greens (e.g., spinach, kale)
1 avocado, sliced
1/4 cup sliced almonds
2 tablespoons tahini
1 tablespoon lemon juice
1 clove garlic, minced
Salt and pepper to taste

Instructions

1. Preheat oven to 400°F (200°C).
2. Place butternut squash cubes and chickpeas on a baking sheet.
3. Drizzle with olive oil, season with salt and pepper, and toss to coat.
4. Roast in the oven for 25 minutes or until squash is tender and chickpeas are crispy.
5. In a small bowl, whisk together tahini, lemon juice, garlic, salt, and pepper to make the dressing.
6. Assemble bowls with mixed greens, roasted squash, chickpeas, avocado slices, and sliced almonds.
7. Drizzle with tahini dressing before serving.
Nutritional Info: Calories: 420, Protein: 14g, Carbohydrates: 50g, Fat: 20g, Fiber: 15g

Veggie and Lentil Shepherd's Pie

Comforting shepherd's pie made with a savory lentil and vegetable filling topped with creamy mashed potatoes.

Preparation Time: 15 minutes
Cooking Time: 40 minutes
Total Time: 55 minutes
Servings: 6

Ingredients

1 cup dried green lentils, rinsed
2 cups vegetable broth
2 tablespoons olive oil
1 onion, diced
2 carrots, diced
2 celery stalks, diced
2 cloves garlic, minced
1 teaspoon dried thyme
1 cup frozen peas
4 cups mashed potatoes
Salt and pepper to taste

Instructions

1. Preheat oven to 375°F (190°C).
2. In a large pot, combine lentils and vegetable broth.
3. Bring to a boil, then reduce heat and simmer for 20 minutes or until lentils are tender.
4. Meanwhile, heat olive oil in a skillet over medium heat. Add onion, carrots, celery, and garlic.
5. Sauté until vegetables are softened.
6. Stir in cooked lentils, thyme, peas, salt, and pepper.
7. Transfer the lentil mixture to a baking dish.
8. Spread mashed potatoes evenly over the top.
9. Bake for 20 minutes or until the mashed potatoes are lightly golden.
10. Serve hot.

Nutritional Info: Calories: 320, Protein: 12g, Carbohydrates: 50g, Fat: 8g, Fiber: 12g

Zucchini Noodles with Avocado Pesto

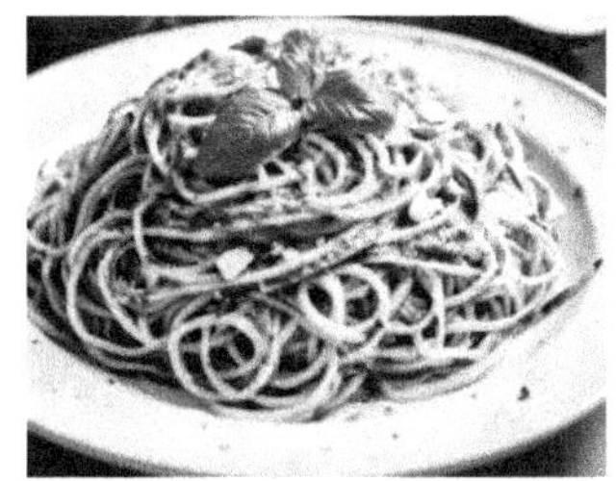

Light and refreshing zucchini noodles tossed in creamy avocado pesto sauce.

Ingredients

2 large zucchini, spiralized into noodles

1 ripe avocado
1 cup fresh basil leaves
1/4 cup pine nuts
2 cloves garlic
Juice of 1 lemon
2 tablespoons olive oil
Salt and pepper to taste

Instructions:

1. In a food processor, combine avocado, basil, pine nuts, garlic, lemon juice, olive oil, salt, and pepper. 2. Blend until smooth and creamy.

3. In a large bowl, toss zucchini noodles with avocado pesto sauce until well coated.

4. Serve immediately, garnished with additional basil leaves if desired.

Nutritional Info: Calories: 280, Protein: 6g, Carbohydrates: 15g, Fat: 22g, Fiber: 8g

Vegan Mushroom Risotto

Creamy and flavorful risotto made with arborio rice and sautéed mushrooms, finished with a touch of nutritional yeast for cheesy flavor.

Preparation Time: 10 minutes
Cooking Time: 30 minutes
Total Time: 40 minutes
Servings: 4

Ingredients

1 cup arborio rice
4 cups vegetable broth
2 tablespoons olive oil
1 onion, diced
2 cloves garlic, minced
8 oz mushrooms, sliced
1/4 cup nutritional yeast
Salt and pepper to taste

Instructions

1. In a large pot, heat vegetable broth over medium heat.

2. In a separate skillet, heat olive oil over medium heat.

3. Add onion and garlic, sauté until translucent.

4. Add mushrooms and cook until browned and tender.

5. Stir in arborio rice and cook for 2-3 minutes until rice is lightly toasted.

6. Add 1/2 cup of vegetable broth at a time, stirring frequently and let the liquid to absorb before adding another one.

7. Continue this process until the rice is creamy and cooked through, about 20-25 minutes.

8. Stir in nutritional yeast, salt, and pepper. Serve hot.

Nutritional Info: Calories: 320, Protein: 8g, Carbohydrates: 50g, Fat: 10g, Fiber: 6g

Cauliflower Fried Rice

Low-carb alternative to traditional fried rice, made with finely chopped cauliflower and mixed vegetables.

Preparation Time: 15 minutes
Cooking Time: 15 minutes
Total Time: 30 minutes
Servings: 4

Ingredients

1 head cauliflower, chopped into florets
2 tablespoons sesame oil
1 onion, diced
2 cloves garlic, minced
1 cup mixed vegetables (such as carrots, peas, bell peppers)
2 tablespoons soy sauce or tamari
2 green onions, sliced
Salt and pepper to taste

Instructions

1. In a food processor, pulse cauliflower florets until they resemble rice grains.
2. Heat sesame oil in a large skillet over medium heat.
3. Add onion and garlic, sauté until fragrant.
4. Add mixed vegetables and cauliflower rice, cook for 5-7 minutes until vegetables are tender.
5. Stir in soy sauce and green onions.
6. Season with salt and pepper.
7. Cook for another 2-3 minutes.
8. Serve hot.

Nutritional Info: Calories: 180, Protein: 6g, Carbohydrates: 25g, Fat: 8g, Fiber: 8g

Lentil and Sweet Potato Curry

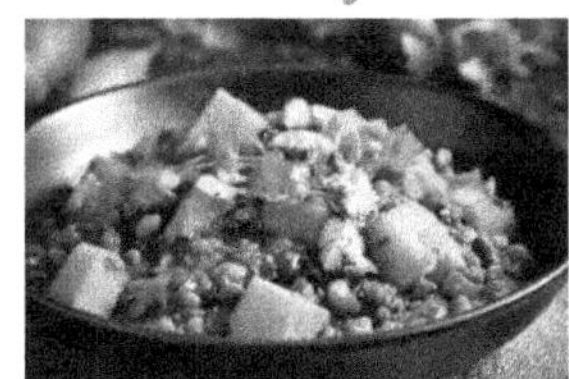

Hearty curry made with lentils, sweet potatoes, and a blend of aromatic spices, served over rice.

Preparation Time: 10 minutes
Cooking Time: 30 minutes
Total Time: 40 minutes
Servings: 4

Ingredients

1 cup dried green lentils, rinsed
2 cups vegetable broth
1 onion, diced
2 cloves garlic, minced
2 teaspoons curry powder

1 teaspoon ground cumin
1/2 teaspoon ground turmeric
2 cups diced sweet potatoes
1 can (14 oz) diced tomatoes
Salt and pepper to taste
Cooked rice for serving

Instructions

1. In a large pot, combine lentils, vegetable broth, onion, garlic, curry powder, cumin, and turmeric. Bring mixture to a boil, then reduce heat to low and simmer for 20 minutes.

2. Add diced sweet potatoes and diced tomatoes to the pot. Continue to simmer for another 10 minutes or until sweet potatoes are tender.

3. Season with salt and pepper. Serve over cooked rice.

Nutritional Info: Calories: 320, Protein: 14g, Carbohydrates: 55g, Fat: 2g, Fiber: 12g

Delicious Mushroom & Spinach Quiche

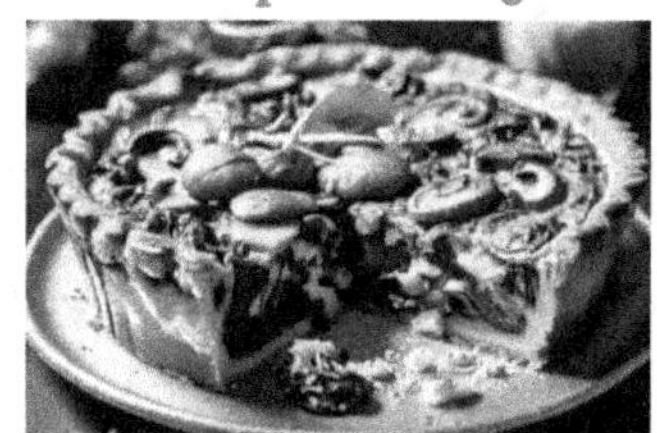

Delicious quiche made with a gluten-free crust filled with sautéed spinach, mushrooms, and a creamy tofu filling.

Preparation Time: 20 minutes
Cooking Time: 40 minutes
Total Time: 1 hour
Serving: 6

Ingredients

For the crust:
1 1/2 cups gluten-free flour
1/2 cup vegan butter, chilled and cubed
3-4 tablespoons ice water
For the filling:
2 cups chopped spinach
1 cup sliced mushrooms
1 onion, diced
2 cloves garlic, minced
1 block (14 oz) firm tofu, drained
1/4 cup nutritional yeast
2 tablespoons olive oil
Salt and pepper to taste

Instructions

1. Preheat oven to 375°F (190°C).

2. In a food processor, pulse gluten-free flour and vegan butter until mixture resembles coarse crumbs.
3. Add ice water, 1 tablespoon at a time, until dough comes together.
4. Press dough into a greased quiche pan or pie dish.
5. In a skillet, heat olive oil over medium heat.
6. Add onion and garlic, sauté until translucent.
7. Add mushrooms and spinach, cook until mushrooms are browned and spinach is wilted.
8. In a food processor, blend tofu, nutritional yeast, salt, and pepper until smooth and creamy.
9. Spread spinach and mushroom mixture over the crust.
10. Pour tofu mixture over the vegetables.
11. Bake for 40 minutes or until set and golden brown. Let it cool slightly before slicing and serving.
Nutritional Info: Calories: 320, Protein: 10g, Carbohydrates: 30g, Fat: 18g, Fiber: 6g

Vegan Pad Thai

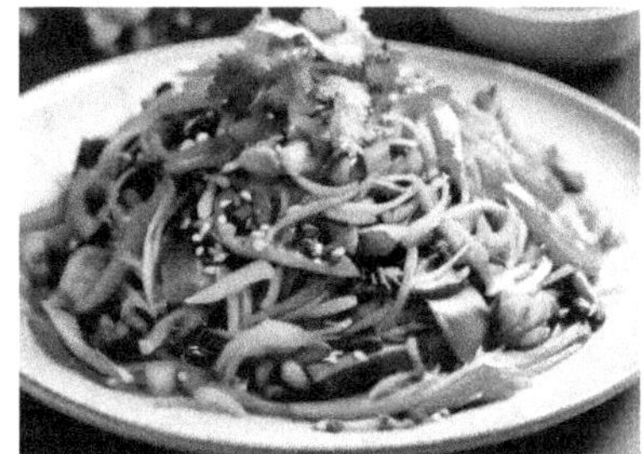

Flavorful and satisfying pad Thai made with rice noodles, tofu, and a tangy tamarind sauce.
Preparation Time: 15 minutes
Cooking Time: 15 minutes
Total Time: 30 minutes
Servings: 4
Ingredients
8 oz rice noodles
1 tablespoon sesame oil
1 block (14 oz) extra firm tofu, drained and cubed
2 cups bean sprouts
1 red bell pepper, thinly sliced
3 green onions, sliced
1/4 cup chopped peanuts
2 tablespoons chopped cilantro
For the sauce:
3 tablespoons tamari
2 tablespoons tamarind paste
1 tablespoon maple syrup
1 tablespoon lime juice
1 clove garlic, minced

1 teaspoon sriracha (optional)
Instructions
1. Cook rice noodles according to package instructions. Drain and set aside.
2. In a small bowl, whisk together all the sauce ingredients. Set aside.
3. Heat sesame oil in a large skillet over medium-high heat.
4. Add tofu cubes and cook until golden brown on all sides.
5. Add bell pepper and green onions, sauté for 2-3 minutes until slightly softened.
6. Add cooked rice noodles and sauce to the skillet.
7. Toss everything together until noodles are well coated.
8. Cook for another 2-3 minutes until heated through.
9. Serve hot, garnished with bean sprouts, chopped peanuts, and cilantro.
Nutritional Info: Calories: 380, Protein: 14g, Carbohydrates: 55g, Fat: 12g, Fiber: 8g

Chickpea and Vegetable Tagine

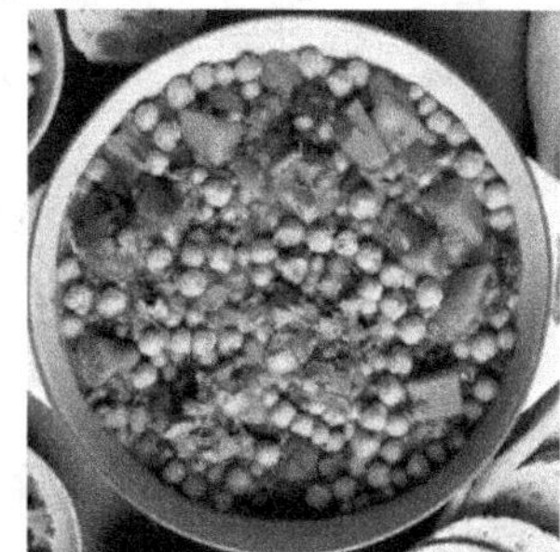

Fragrant Moroccan-inspired stew made with chickpeas, vegetables, and a blend of aromatic spices.
Preparation Time: 15 minutes
Cooking Time: 30 minutes
Total Time: 45 minutes
Servings: 4
Ingredients
1 tablespoon olive oil
1 onion, diced
2 cloves garlic, minced
1 teaspoon ground cumin
1 teaspoon ground coriander
1/2 teaspoon ground cinnamon
1/4 teaspoon ground ginger
1 can (15 oz) chickpeas, drained and rinsed
2 cups diced tomatoes
1 cup vegetable broth
2 cups diced mixed vegetables (e.g., carrots, zucchini, bell peppers)
Salt and pepper to taste
Cooked couscous for serving
Instructions
1. Heat the oil in a large pot over medium heat.
2. Add onion and garlic, let it sauté until softened.

3. Stir in ground cumin, coriander, cinnamon, and ginger.
4. Add chickpeas, diced tomatoes, vegetable broth, and mixed vegetables to the pot.
5. Bring to a simmer and cook for 20-25 minutes until vegetables are tender and flavors have melded together.
6. Season with salt and pepper.
7. Serve hot over cooked couscous.
Nutritional Info: Calories: 340, Protein: 12g, Carbohydrates: 50g, Fat: 8g, Fiber: 10g

Vegan Lentil Sloppy Joes

A vegan twist on a classic comfort food, made with hearty lentils simmered in a savory tomato sauce, served on gluten-free buns.
Preparation Time: 15 minutes
Cooking Time: 30 minutes
Total Time: 45 minutes
Servings: 4
Ingredients
1 cup dried green lentils, rinsed
3 cups vegetable broth
1 tablespoon olive oil
1 onion, diced
2 cloves garlic, minced
1 bell pepper, diced
1 can (14 oz) diced tomatoes
2 tablespoons tomato paste
2 tablespoons maple syrup
1 tablespoon apple cider vinegar
1 teaspoon chili powder
Salt and pepper to taste
Gluten-free hamburger buns for serving
Instructions
1. In a large pot, combine lentils and vegetable broth.
2. Bring to a boil, then reduce heat and simmer for 20-25 minutes until lentils are tender and most of the liquid has been absorbed.
3. Meanwhile, heat olive oil in a skillet over medium heat.
4. Add onion, garlic, and bell pepper, sauté until softened.
5. Stir in diced tomatoes, tomato paste, maple syrup, apple cider vinegar, chili powder, salt, and pepper.
6. Simmer for 5-10 minutes until flavors are well combined.
7. Add cooked lentils to the skillet and stir to coat in the sauce.
8. Serve hot on gluten-free hamburger buns.
Nutritional Info: Calories: 320, Protein: 12g, Carbohydrates: 50g, Fat: 8g, Fiber: 10g

Millet Salad with Almonds and Carrots

A refreshing salad packed with nutrients and texture.
Preparation Time: 15 minutes

Cooking Time: 20 minutes
Total Time: 35 minutes
Servings: 2
Ingredients
1 cup cooked millet
1/2 cup shredded carrots
1/4 cup sliced almonds
1 tablespoon flaxseeds
2 cups mixed greens
Salt and pepper to taste

Instructions
1. In a large bowl, combine cooked millet, shredded carrots, sliced almonds, and flaxseeds.
2. Add mixed greens and toss gently.
3. Season with salt and pepper to taste.
4. Serve immediately.
Nutritional Info: Calories: 280, Protein: 8g, Carbohydrates: 40g, Fat: 10g, Fiber: 8g

Apple Chia Seed Pudding

A creamy and satisfying pudding perfect for a quick lunch.
Preparation Time: 10 minutes (plus chilling time)
Cooking Time: 0 minutes
Total Time: 10 minutes (plus chilling time)
Servings: 2
Ingredients
2 medium apples, peeled and diced
2 tablespoons chia seeds
1 cup almond milk
1 teaspoon cinnamon
1 tablespoon maple syrup (optional)

Instructions
1. In a blender, combine diced apples, chia seeds, almond milk, cinnamon, and maple syrup (if using).
2. Blend until smooth.
3. Pour the mixture into a bowl and refrigerate for at least 2 hours or until set.
4. Serve chilled.
Nutritional Info: Calories: 180, Protein: 4g, Carbohydrates: 30g, Fat: 6g, Fiber: 10g

Almond Butter and Apple Sandwich

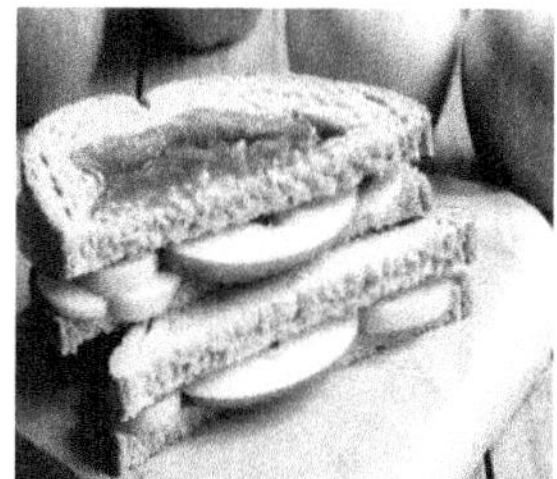

A satisfying sandwich with a sweet and nutty flavor.
Preparation Time: 5 minutes
Cooking Time: 0 minutes
Total Time: 5 minutes
Servings: 1
Ingredients:
2 slices gluten-free bread
2 tablespoons almond butter
1/2 apple, thinly sliced
Instructions
1. Spread almond butter evenly onto one slice of bread.
2. Arrange thinly sliced apple on top of the almond butter.
3. Place the remaining slice of bread on top to form a sandwich.
4. Slice in half and serve.
Nutritional Info: Calories: 320, Protein: 8g, Carbohydrates: 35g, Fat: 18g, Fiber: 6g

Millet Stuffed Bell Peppers

Colorful bell peppers stuffed with hearty millet and vegetable filling.
Preparation Time: 15 minutes
Cooking Time: 40 minutes
Total Time: 55 minutes
Servings: 4
Ingredients
1 cup cooked millet
4 bell peppers, halved and seeds removed
1 small onion, diced
2 cloves garlic, minced
1 cup diced tomatoes
1/2 cup vegetable broth
1 teaspoon dried oregano
Salt and pepper to taste
Instructions
1. Preheat the oven to 375°F (190°C).
2. Heat the oil in a medium skillet, over medium heat.
3. Add diced onion and minced garlic, sauté until softened.
4. Stir in cooked millet, diced tomatoes, vegetable broth, dried oregano, salt, and pepper. Cook for 5 minutes.

5. Stuff each halved bell pepper with the millet mixture.
6. Place stuffed bell peppers in a baking dish, cover with foil, and bake for 30 minutes.
7. Remove foil and bake for an additional 10 minutes, or until peppers are tender.
8. Serve hot.
Nutritional Info: Calories: 220, Protein: 6g, Carbohydrates: 40g, Fat: 4g, Fiber: 8g

Apple and Almond Quinoa Salad

A protein-packed salad with a sweet and crunchy twist.
Preparation Time: 15 minutes
Cooking Time: 15 minutes
Total Time: 30 minutes
Servings: 2
Ingredients
1 cup cooked quinoa
1/2 apple, diced
1/4 cup sliced almonds
2 cups baby spinach
2 tablespoons apple cider vinegar
1 tablespoon olive oil
1 teaspoon Dijon mustard
Salt and pepper to taste
Instructions
1. In a large bowl, combine cooked quinoa, diced apple, sliced almonds, and baby spinach.
2. In a small bowl, whisk together apple cider vinegar, olive oil, Dijon mustard, salt, and pepper to make the dressing.
3. Pour the dressing over the salad and toss to coat evenly.
4. Serve chilled or at room temperature.
Nutritional Info: Calories: 280, Protein: 8g, Carbohydrates: 35g, Fat: 12g, Fiber: 6g

Carrot and Chia Seed Muffins

Moist and fluffy muffins packed with carrots and chia seeds.
Preparation Time: 15 minutes
Cooking Time: 20 minutes
Total Time: 35 minutes
Servings: 6
Ingredients
1 cup gluten-free flour
1/2 cup almond flour
1/4 cup chia seeds
1 teaspoon baking powder
1/2 teaspoon baking soda
1/4 teaspoon salt
1/2 cup unsweetened applesauce
1/4 cup maple syrup

1/4 cup almond milk
2 tablespoons coconut oil, melted
1 teaspoon vanilla extract
1 cup grated carrots
Instructions
1. Preheat the oven to 375°F (190°C). Line a muffin tin with paper liners.
2. In a large bowl, whisk together gluten-free flour, almond flour, chia seeds, baking powder, baking soda, and salt.
3. In another bowl, mix together applesauce, maple syrup, almond milk, coconut oil, and vanilla extract.
4. Pour the wet ingredients into the dry ingredients and stir until combined. Fold in grated carrots.
5. Divide the batter evenly among the muffin cups.
6. Bake for 18-20 minutes, or until a toothpick inserted into the center comes out clean.
7. Allow the muffins to cool in the pan for 5 minutes before transferring to a wire rack to cool completely.
Nutritional Info: Calories: 220, Protein: 5g, Carbohydrates: 30g, Fat: 10g, Fiber: 6g

Almond Crusted Tofu with Carrot Ginger Sauce

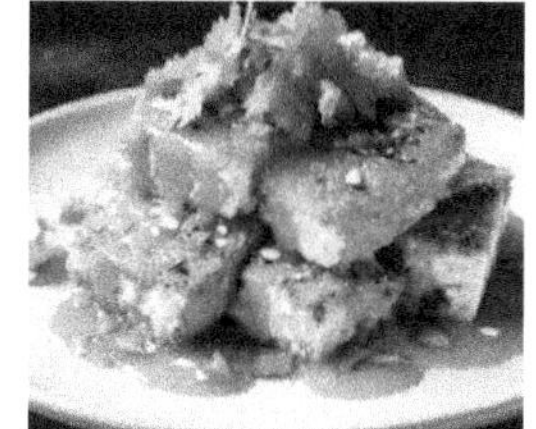

Crispy almond-crusted tofu served with a flavorful carrot ginger sauce.
Preparation Time: 20 minutes
Cooking Time: 20 minutes
Total Time: 40 minutes
Servings: 2
Ingredients
1 block tofu, pressed and sliced
1/4 cup almond meal
1/4 teaspoon garlic powder
1/4 teaspoon onion powder
Salt and pepper to taste
2 tablespoons olive oil
1 cup shredded carrots
1 tablespoon grated ginger
2 cloves garlic, minced
1 tablespoon tamari
1 tablespoon rice vinegar
1 tablespoon maple syrup
1/4 cup vegetable broth

Instructions
1. Preheat the oven to 400°F (200°C). Line a baking sheet with parchment paper.
2. In a shallow dish, combine almond meal, garlic powder, onion powder, salt, and pepper.
3. Dip each tofu slice into the almond mixture, coating evenly on both sides. Place on the prepared baking sheet.
4. Drizzle olive oil over the tofu slices. Bake for 20 minutes, flipping halfway through, until golden brown and crispy.
5. Meanwhile, prepare the carrot ginger sauce.
6. In a skillet, heat olive oil over medium heat. Add shredded carrots, grated ginger, and minced garlic.
7. Sauté for 5 minutes.
8. Stir in tamari, rice vinegar, maple syrup, and vegetable broth.
9. Cook for another 5 minutes, until the carrots are tender.
10. Serve the almond-crusted tofu with the carrot ginger sauce.
Nutritional Info: Calories: 320, Protein: 12g, Carbohydrates: 25g, Fat: 18g, Fiber: 6g

Chia Seed Veggie Wraps

Fresh and light veggie wraps with a chia seed twist.
Preparation Time: 15 minutes
Cooking Time: 0 minutes
Total Time: 15 minutes
Servings: 2
Ingredients
4 large collard green leaves
1/2 cup hummus
1/2 cup shredded carrots
1/2 cucumber, julienned
1/2 bell pepper, thinly sliced
2 tablespoons chia seeds
Instructions
1. Lay the collard green leaves flat on a cutting board. Trim the tough stem.
2. Spread a layer of hummus onto each collard green leaf.
3. Layer shredded carrots, julienned cucumber, and sliced bell pepper on top of the hummus.
4. Sprinkle chia seeds over the veggies.
5. Roll up the collard green leaves tightly, tucking in the sides as you go.
6. Slice the wraps in half and serve.
Nutritional Info: Calories: 180, Protein: 6g, Carbohydrates: 25g, Fat: 8g, Fiber: 10g

SOUP

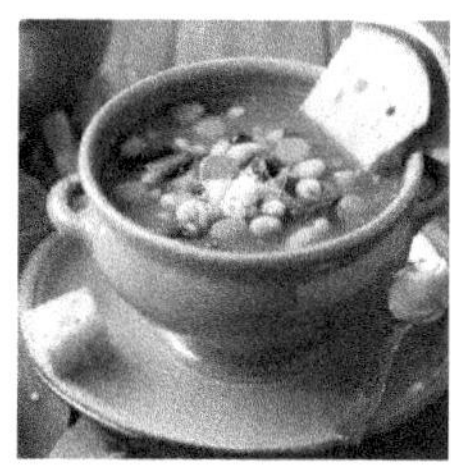

Classic Minestrone Soup

A hearty Italian soup loaded with vegetables, beans, and pasta in a flavorful tomato broth.
Preparation Time: 15 minutes
Cooking Time: 30 minutes
Total Time: 45 minutes
Servings: 6

Ingredients
2 tablespoons olive oil
1 onion, diced
2 carrots, diced
2 celery stalks, diced
3 cloves garlic, minced
1 can (15 oz) diced tomatoes
6 cups vegetable broth
1 can (15 oz) cannellini beans, drained and rinsed
1 cup gluten-free pasta (such as rice or quinoa pasta)
2 cups chopped spinach or kale
1 teaspoon dried oregano
1 teaspoon dried basil
Salt and pepper to taste
Fresh parsley for garnish

Instructions
1. Heat olive oil in a large pot over medium heat.
2. Add onion, celery and carrots. Cook until softened.
3. Add the garlic and cook until fragrant.
4. Stir in diced tomatoes, vegetable broth, cannellini beans, gluten-free pasta, dried oregano, and dried basil.
5. Bring to a boil, then reduce heat and simmer for 15-20 minutes, or until pasta is tender.
6. Stir in chopped spinach or kale and cook until wilted.
7. Season with salt and pepper to taste.
8. Serve hot, garnished with fresh parsley.

Nutritional Info: Calories: 220, Protein: 8g, Carbohydrates: 35g, Fat: 6g, Fiber: 8g

Curried Butternut Squash Soup

Creamy butternut squash soup infused with warm curry spices, perfect for a cozy night in.
Preparation Time: 15 minutes

Cooking Time: 40 minutes
Total Time: 55 minutes
Servings: 4

Ingredients

1 medium butternut squash, peeled, seeded, and cubed
1 onion, chopped
2 cloves garlic, minced
1 tablespoon olive oil
2 teaspoons curry powder
1/2 teaspoon ground cumin
1/4 teaspoon ground cinnamon
4 cups vegetable broth
Salt and pepper to taste
Coconut milk for garnish (optional)
Fresh cilantro for garnish

Instructions

1. In a medium pot, heat the oil over medium heat.
2. Add chopped onion and minced garlic. Cook until softened.
3. Add cubed butternut squash to the pot, along with curry powder, ground cumin, and ground cinnamon.
4. Stir to coat the squash with the spices.
5. Pour in vegetable broth and bring to a boil.
6. Reduce heat and simmer for 20-25 minutes, or until the squash is tender.
7. Use an immersion blender to puree the soup until smooth. Alternatively, carefully transfer the soup to a blender and blend in batches until smooth.
8. Season the soup with salt and pepper to taste.
9. Garnished with a swirl of coconut milk and fresh cilantro if you want and Serve ho enjoy!

Nutritional Info: Calories: 180, Protein: 3g, Carbohydrates: 30g, Fat: 7g, Fiber: 6g

Vegan Lentil Soup

Hearty and comforting lentil soup packed with vegetables and aromatic spices.
Preparation Time: 15 minutes
Cooking Time: 40 minutes
Total Time: 55 minutes
Servings: 6

Ingredients

1 cup dried green lentils, rinsed
1 onion, diced
2 carrots, diced
2 celery stalks, diced
3 cloves garlic, minced
1 can (14 oz) diced tomatoes
6 cups vegetable broth
1 teaspoon ground cumin
1 teaspoon ground coriander

1/2 teaspoon smoked paprika
Salt and pepper to taste
2 cups chopped spinach or kale
Juice of 1 lemon
Fresh parsley for garnish

Instructions

1. In a large soup pot, heat the oil over medium heat.
2. Add diced onion, carrots, and celery. Cook until vegetables are softened.
3. Add minced garlic, ground cumin, ground coriander, smoked paprika, salt, and pepper.
4. Cook for another minute until fragrant.
5. Stir in dried lentils, diced tomatoes, and vegetable broth.
6. Bring to a boil, then reduce heat and simmer for 30-35 minutes, or until lentils are tender.
7. Add chopped spinach or kale and lemon juice. Cook for an additional 5 minutes.
8. Taste and adjust seasoning if needed.
9. Serve hot, garnished with fresh parsley.

Nutritional Info: Calories: 220, Protein: 10g, Carbohydrates: 35g, Fat: 5g, Fiber: 12g

Carrot and Flaxseed Soup

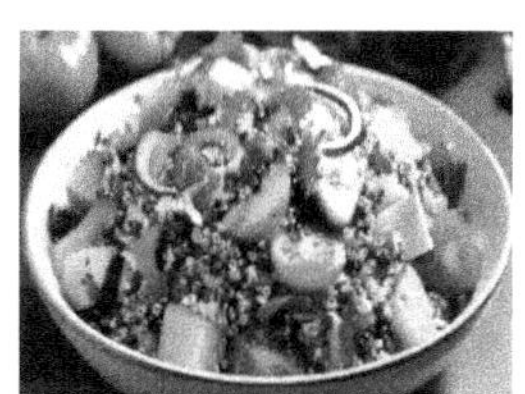

A comforting and nutritious soup perfect for main meal.
Preparation Time: 10 minutes
Cooking Time: 25 minutes
Total Time: 35 minutes
Servings: 4

Ingredients

4 large carrots, peeled and chopped
1 onion, chopped
2 cloves garlic, minced
1 tablespoon olive oil
4 cups vegetable broth
2 tablespoons ground flaxseeds
Salt and pepper to taste

Instructions

1. Heat the oil in a large soup pot over medium heat.
2. Add the onion and garlic to the heated oil and let sauté until softened.
3. Add chopped carrots and vegetable broth.
4. Bring to a boil, then reduce heat to low and simmer for about 20 minutes or until carrots are tender.
5. Use an immersion blender to blend the soup until smooth.

6. Stir in ground flaxseeds and season with salt and pepper to taste.
7. Serve hot.
Nutritional Info: Calories: 150, Protein: 3g, Carbohydrates: 20g, Fat: 8g, Fiber: 6g

Tomato Basil Soup

A classic tomato soup infused with the fresh flavor of basil, perfect for a comforting meal.
Preparation Time: 10 minutes
Cooking Time: 30 minutes
Total Time: 40 minutes
Servings: 4
Ingredients
2 tablespoons olive oil
1 onion, diced
2 cloves garlic, minced
1 can (28 oz) crushed tomatoes
4 cups vegetable broth
1/4 cup chopped fresh basil leaves
1 teaspoon dried oregano
Salt and pepper to taste
Optional: coconut cream for garnish
Instructions
1. Heat the oil in a large soup pot over medium heat.
2. Add diced onion and minced garlic. Cook until softened.
3. Stir in crushed tomatoes, vegetable broth, chopped fresh basil, and dried oregano.
4. Bring to a boil, then reduce heat and simmer for 20-25 minutes.
5. Use an immersion blender to blend the soup until smooth or transfer the soup to a blender and blend until smooth.
6. Season with salt and pepper to taste.
7. Serve hot, garnished with a drizzle of coconut cream and additional fresh basil if desired.
Nutritional Info: Calories: 160, Protein: 3g, Carbohydrates: 20g, Fat: 9g, Fiber: 5g

Lentil Vegetable Soup

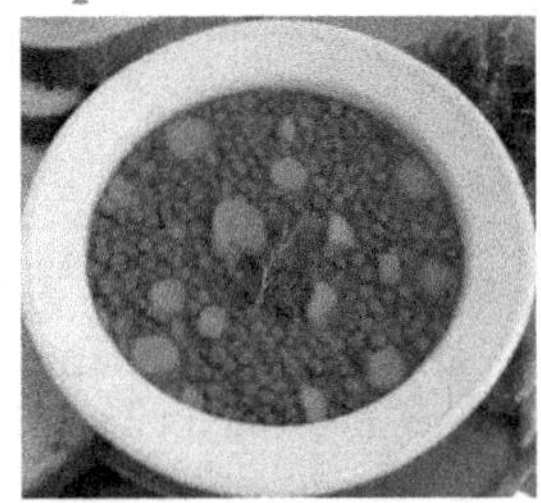

Hearty lentil soup packed with vegetables and aromatic spices, a comforting and nutritious meal.
Preparation Time: 15 minutes
Cooking Time: 40 minutes
Total Time: 55 minutes

Servings: 6
Ingredients
1 cup dried brown or green lentils, rinsed
1 onion, diced
2 carrots, diced
2 celery stalks, diced
3 cloves garlic, minced
1 can (14 oz) diced tomatoes
6 cups vegetable broth
1 teaspoon ground cumin
1 teaspoon paprika
1/2 teaspoon dried thyme
Salt and pepper to taste
Fresh parsley for garnish
Instructions
1. In a large pot, combine vegetable broth, diced tomatoes, diced onion, diced carrots, diced celery, minced garlic, lentils, ground cumin, paprika, dried thyme, salt, and pepper.
2. Bring the soup to a boil over medium-high heat.
3. Once boiling, reduce the heat to low and let the soup simmer for 30-35 minutes, or until the lentils and vegetables are tender.
4. Adjust seasoning with salt and pepper if needed.
5. Serve hot, garnished with fresh parsley.
Nutritional Info: Calories: 220, Protein: 12g, Carbohydrates: 35g, Fat: 2g, Fiber: 10g

Coconut Curry Lentil Soup

Creamy coconut curry lentil soup with a hint of spice, packed with protein and flavor.
Preparation Time: 15 minutes
Cooking Time: 35 minutes
Total Time: 50 minutes
Servings: 4
Ingredients
1 cup dried red lentils, rinsed
1 onion, diced
2 carrots, diced
2 celery stalks, diced
3 cloves garlic, minced
1 tablespoon curry powder
1 can (14 oz) coconut milk
4 cups vegetable broth
1 tablespoon coconut oil
Salt and pepper to taste
Fresh cilantro for garnish
Instructions
1. In a large pot, heat coconut oil over medium heat.
2. Add diced onion, carrots, celery, and minced garlic. Cook until softened.

3. Stir in curry powder and cook for another minute until fragrant.
4. Add dried red lentils, coconut milk, and vegetable broth to the pot.
5. Bring to a boil, then reduce heat and simmer for 25-30 minutes, or until lentils are tender.
6. Use an immersion blender to puree the soup until smooth. Alternatively, carefully transfer the soup to a blender and blend until smooth.
7. Season with salt and pepper to taste.
8. Serve hot, garnished with fresh cilantro.
Nutritional Info: Calories: 280, Protein: 15g, Carbohydrates: 35g, Fat: 10g, Fiber: 8g

Vegetable Quinoa Soup

Nutritious vegetable soup with quinoa, packed with protein, fiber, and vitamins.
Preparation Time: 15 minutes
Cooking Time: 25 minutes
Total Time: 40 minutes
Servings: 4
Ingredients
1 tablespoon olive oil
1 onion, diced
2 carrots, diced
2 celery stalks, diced
3 cloves garlic, minced
1 can (14 oz) diced tomatoes
4 cups vegetable broth
1/2 cup quinoa, rinsed
2 cups chopped spinach or kale
1 teaspoon dried thyme
Salt and pepper to taste
Fresh parsley for garnish
Instructions
1. Heat the oil large pot over medium heat
2. Add diced onion, carrots, celery, and minced garlic. Cook until softened.
3. Stir in diced tomatoes, vegetable broth, quinoa, and dried thyme.
4. Bring to a boil, then reduce heat and simmer for 15-20 minutes, or until quinoa is cooked.
5. Stir in chopped spinach or kale and cook until wilted.
6. Season the soup with salt and pepper to taste.
7. Serve hot, garnished with fresh parsley.
Nutritional Info: Calories: 240, Protein: 8g, Carbohydrates: 35g, Fat: 6g, Fiber: 8g

Mushroom Almond Flour Soup

A rich and creamy soup featuring the earthy flavor of mushrooms and the nuttiness of almond flour.
Preparation Time: 10 minutes
Cooking Time: 25 minutes
Total Time: 35 minutes

Servings Size: 4

Ingredients

2 cups sliced mushrooms

1 onion, diced

2 cloves garlic, minced

1/4 cup almond flour

4 cups vegetable broth

1/2 cup coconut milk

1 tablespoon olive oil

Salt and pepper to taste

Instructions

1. Heat the oil in a a soup pot over medium heat.
2. Add onion and garlic to the heated oil, sauté until softened.
3. Add the mushrooms and cook until they release their moisture.
4. Sprinkle almond flour over the mushrooms, stirring to coat evenly.
5. Pour in vegetable broth and coconut milk. Bring to a simmer.
6. Simmer for 15-20 minutes until the soup thickens slightly.
7. Season with salt and pepper before serving.

Nutritional Info: Calories: 240, Protein: 5g, Carbohydrates: 15g, Fat: 15g, Fiber: 3g

Quinoa Carrot Ginger Soup

A comforting and aromatic soup featuring the wholesome goodness of quinoa and the warmth of ginger.

Preparation Time: 15 minutes

Cooking Time: 25 minutes

Total Time: 40 minutes

Servings: 4

Ingredients

1 cup quinoa, rinsed

4 cups vegetable broth

4 large carrots, peeled and chopped

1 onion, diced

2 cloves garlic, minced

1-inch piece of ginger, grated

1 tablespoon olive oil

Salt and pepper to taste

Instructions

1. Heat olive oil in a pot over medium heat.
2. Add onion, garlic, and ginger, sauté until fragrant.
3. Add chopped carrots and cook for a few minutes.
4. Stir in quinoa and vegetable broth. Bring to a boil.
5. Reduce heat, cover, and simmer for 20-25 minutes until quinoa and carrots are tender.
6. Use an immersion blender or transfer to a blender to puree until smooth.
7. Season with salt and pepper before serving.

Nutritional Info: Calories: 250, Protein: 7g, Carbohydrates: 40g, Fat: 5g, Fiber: 6g

Spicy Black Bean Soup

Flavorful black bean soup with a kick of spice, perfect for a satisfying meal.
Preparation Time: 15 minutes
Cooking Time: 30 minutes
Total Time: 45 minutes
Servings: 4
Ingredients
2 tablespoons olive oil
1 onion, diced
2 cloves garlic, minced
1 red bell pepper, diced
1 jalapeño pepper, seeded and minced
2 teaspoons ground cumin
1 teaspoon chili powder
1/2 teaspoon smoked paprika
2 cans black beans (15 oz. each), drained and rinsed
4 cups vegetable broth
1 can (14 oz) diced tomatoes
Juice of 1 lime
Salt and pepper to taste
Fresh cilantro for garnish
Instructions
1. Heat the oil in a large soup pot over medium heat.
2. Add diced onion, minced garlic, diced red bell pepper, and minced jalapeño pepper. Cook until softened.
3. Stir in ground cumin, chili powder, and smoked paprika.
4. Cook for another minute until fragrant.
5. Add black beans, vegetable broth, and diced tomatoes to the pot.
6. Bring to a boil, then reduce to low heat and simmer for about 25 minutes.
7. Blend the soup with immersion blender until smooth or transfer the soup to a blender and blend until smooth.
8. Stir in lime juice and season with salt and pepper to taste.
9. Serve hot, garnished with fresh cilantro.
Nutritional Info: Calories: 230, Protein: 10g, Carbohydrates: 35g, Fat: 7g, Fiber: 10g

Roasted Vegetable Soup

Rich and flavorful soup made with roasted vegetables, blended to perfection for a comforting meal.
Preparation Time: 15 minutes
Cooking Time: 45 minutes
Total Time: 1 hour
Servings: 4
Ingredients
1 small butternut squash, peeled, seeded, and cubed
2 carrots, peeled and chopped
2 parsnips, peeled and chopped
1 onion, chopped

3 cloves garlic, minced
2 tablespoons olive oil
4 cups vegetable broth
1 teaspoon dried thyme
Salt and pepper to taste
Fresh parsley for garnish

Instructio3.ns

1. Preheat the oven to 400°F (200°C).
2. Place cubed butternut squash, chopped carrots, chopped parsnips, chopped onion, and minced garlic on a baking sheet.
3. Drizzle the mixture with oil and toss to coat.
4. Roast vegetables in the preheated oven for 25-30 minutes, or until tender and caramelized.
5. In a large pot, combine roasted vegetables, vegetable broth, and dried thyme.
6. Bring to a boil, then reduce heat to low and simmer for about 15 minutes.
7. Remove the soup from the heat and transfer to a blender and blend until smooth, you can also blend with an immersion blender.
8. Season with salt and pepper to taste.
9. Serve hot, garnished with fresh parsley.

Nutritional Info: Calories: 210, Protein: 5g, Carbohydrates: 30g, Fat: 9g, Fiber: 8g

Thai Coconut Vegetable Soup

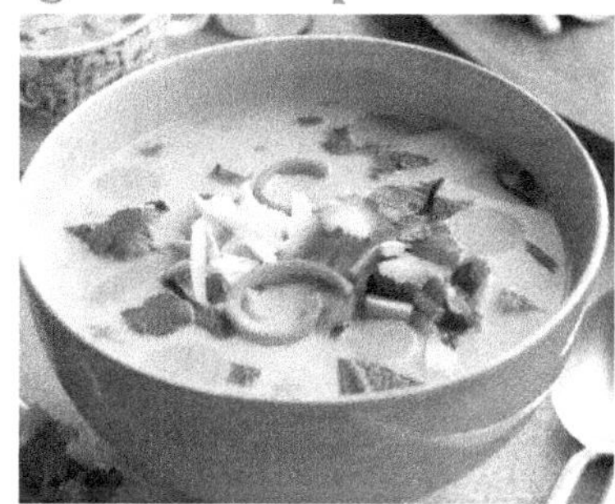

A creamy and aromatic Thai-inspired soup with coconut milk, lemongrass, and fresh vegetables.

Preparation Time: 20 minutes
Cooking Time: 25 minutes
Total Time: 45 minutes
Servings: 4

Ingredients

1 tablespoon coconut oil
1 onion, diced
2 cloves garlic, minced
1 red bell pepper, thinly sliced
1 carrot, thinly sliced
1 zucchini, diced
1 can (14 oz) coconut milk
4 cups vegetable broth

2 tablespoons soy sauce or tamari
1 tablespoon lime juice
1 tablespoon brown sugar or coconut sugar
1 stalk lemongrass, bruised
2 tablespoons chopped fresh cilantro
Salt and pepper to taste

Instructions

1. In a large soup pot, heat oil over medium heat.
2. Add diced onion and minced garlic. Cook until softened.
3. Add thinly sliced red bell pepper, thinly sliced carrot, and diced zucchini to the pot.
4. Cook for 5-7 minutes, or until vegetables are slightly softened.
5. Stir in coconut milk, vegetable broth, soy sauce or tamari, lime juice, brown sugar or coconut sugar, and bruised lemongrass stalk.
6. Bring to a simmer and cook for 15-20 minutes.
7. Remove the lemongrass stalk from the soup and discard.
8. Season the soup with salt and pepper to taste.
9. Serve hot, garnished with chopped fresh cilantro.

Nutritional Info: Calories: 290, Protein: 5g, Carbohydrates: 20g, Fat: 15g, Fiber: 5g

Potato Leek Soup

A comforting and creamy soup made with potatoes, leeks, and vegetable broth, perfect for a cozy meal.

Preparation Time: 15 minutes
Cooking Time: 30 minutes
Total Time: 45 minutes
Servings: 4

Ingredients

2 tablespoons olive oil
2 leeks, white and light green parts only, finely sliced
3 cloves garlic, minced
3 large potatoes, peeled and diced
4 cups vegetable broth
1/2 cup unsweetened almond milk
Salt and pepper to taste
Fresh chives for garnish

Instructions

1. In a large soup pot, heat oil over medium-high heat.
2. Add thinly sliced leeks and minced garlic. Cook until softened.
3. Add diced potatoes and vegetable broth to the pot.
4. Bring to a boil, then reduce heat and simmer for 20-25 minutes, or until potatoes are tender.
5. Use an immersion blender to blend the soup until smooth or transfer the soup to a blender and blend until smooth.
6. Stir in unsweetened almond milk and heat through.
7. Season with salt and pepper to taste.

8. Serve hot, garnished with fresh chives.
Nutritional Info: Calories: 220, Protein: 5g, Carbohydrates: 30g, Fat: 8g, Fiber: 5g

Black Bean and Sweet Potato Soup

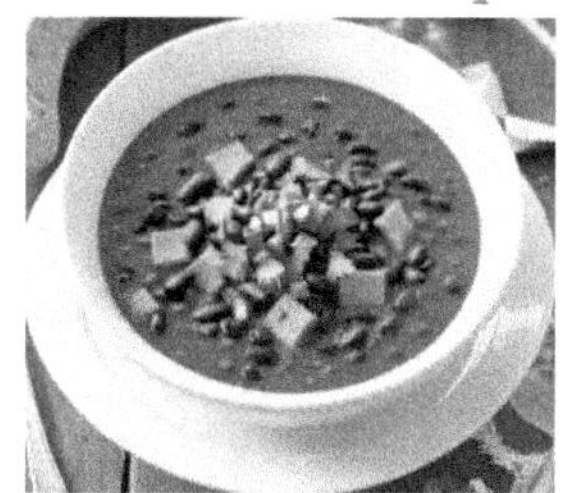

A flavorful and hearty soup made with black beans, sweet potatoes, and spices, perfect for a satisfying meal.
Preparation Time: 20 minutes
Cooking Time: 35 minutes
Total Time: 55 minutes
Servings: 4
Ingredients
1 tablespoon olive oil
1 onion, diced
2 cloves garlic, minced
1 teaspoon ground cumin
1/2 teaspoon chili powder
1/2 teaspoon smoked paprika
2 sweet potatoes, peeled and diced
2 cans black beans (15 oz. each), drained and rinsed
4 cups vegetable broth
1 can (14 oz) diced tomatoes
Salt and pepper to taste
Fresh cilantro for garnish
Instructions
1. Heat the olive oil in a large soup pot over medium heat.
2. Add diced onion and minced garlic. Cook until softened.
3. Stir in ground cumin, chili powder, and smoked paprika.
4. Cook for another minute until fragrant.
5. Add diced sweet potatoes, black beans, vegetable broth, and diced tomatoes to the pot.
6. Bring to a boil, then reduce heat and simmer for 25-30 minutes, or until sweet potatoes are tender.
7. Use an immersion blender to puree a portion of the soup, leaving some chunks of sweet potato and black beans for texture.
8. Season with salt and pepper to taste.
9. Serve hot, garnished with fresh cilantro.
Nutritional Info: Calories: 280, Protein: 10g, Carbohydrates: 45g, Fat: 5g, Fiber: 12g

Mushroom Barley Soup

A hearty and comforting soup made with mushrooms, barley, and aromatic herbs, perfect for a nourishing meal.

Preparation Time: 15 minutes
Cooking Time: 45 minutes
Total Time: 1 hour
Servings: 6

Ingredients

1 tablespoon olive oil
1 onion, diced
2 carrots, diced
2 celery stalks, diced
3 cloves garlic, minced
8 oz cremini mushrooms, sliced
1 cup pearl barley
6 cups vegetable broth
1 teaspoon dried thyme
1 bay leaf
Salt and pepper to taste
Fresh parsley for garnish

Instructions

1. In a large soup pot, heat the oil over medium heat.
3. Add minced garlic and sliced cremini mushrooms to the pot.
4. Cook until mushrooms are golden. Enjoy!

Nutritional Info: Calories: 280, Protein: 8g, Carbohydrates: 45g, Fat: 5g, Fiber: 8g

Italian Wedding Soup

A comforting soup featuring mini meatballs, vegetables, and pasta in a flavorful broth, perfect for a cozy meal.

Preparation Time: 20 minutes
Cooking Time: 30 minutes
Total Time: 50 minutes
Servings: 6

Ingredients

For the meatballs:
1/2 lb ground turkey or beef
1/4 cup gluten-free breadcrumbs
1/4 cup grated Parmesan cheese
1 egg
1 tablespoon chopped fresh parsley
1/2 teaspoon garlic powder
Salt and pepper to taste
For the soup:
1 tablespoon olive oil
1 onion, diced
2 carrots, diced

2 celery stalks, diced
3 cloves garlic, minced
8 cups chicken or vegetable broth
1 cup gluten-free pasta (such as mini shells or ditalini)
2 cups baby spinach or kale
Salt and pepper to taste
Fresh parsley for garnish

Instructions

1. In a bowl, combine ground turkey or beef, gluten-free breadcrumbs, grated Parmesan cheese, egg, chopped fresh parsley, garlic powder, salt, and pepper.
2. Mix until well combined, then shape into small meatballs.
3. In a large pot, heat olive oil over medium heat.
4. Add diced onion, carrots, and celery. Cook until softened.
5. Add minced garlic to the pot and cook until fragrant.
6. Pour in chicken or vegetable broth and bring to a boil.
7. Add gluten-free pasta and meatballs to the pot.
8. Cook for 8-10 minutes, or until pasta is tender and meatballs are cooked through.
9. Stir in baby spinach or kale and cook until wilted.
10. Season with salt and pepper to taste.
11. Serve hot, garnished with fresh parsley.

Nutritional Info: Calories: 320, Protein: 20g, Carbohydrates: 25g, Fat: 15g, Fiber: 5g

Creamy Cauliflower Soup

A velvety smooth soup made with cauliflower, garlic, and onions, blended to perfection for a comforting meal.

Preparation Time: 15 minutes
Cooking Time: 25 minutes
Total Time: 40 minutes
Servings: 4

Ingredients

1 head cauliflower, chopped into florets
1 onion, chopped
3 cloves garlic, minced
2 tablespoons olive oil
4 cups vegetable broth
1/2 cup unsweetened almond milk
Salt and pepper to taste
Fresh chives for garnish

Instructions

1. In a large pot, heat olive oil over medium heat.
2. Add chopped onion and minced garlic. Cook until softened.
3. Add chopped cauliflower florets to the pot and cook for 5 minutes.
4. Pour in vegetable broth and bring to a boil.
5. Reduce heat and simmer for 15-20 minutes, or until cauliflower is tender.

6. Use an immersion blender to puree the soup until smooth. Alternatively, carefully transfer the soup to a blender and blend until smooth.
7. Stir in unsweetened almond milk and heat through.
8. Season with salt and pepper to taste.
9. Serve hot, garnished with fresh chives.
Nutritional Info: Calories: 180, Protein: 5g, Carbohydrates: 20g, Fat: 10g, Fiber: 6g

Millet Mushroom Soup

A creamy and comforting soup featuring earthy mushrooms and nutty millet.
Preparation Time: 10 minutes
Cooking Time: 30 minutes
Total Time: 40 minutes
Servings: 4
Ingredients
1 cup millet, rinsed
4 cups vegetable broth
1 onion, diced
2 cloves garlic, minced
2 cups chopped mushrooms
1 teaspoon dried thyme
1 bay leaf
Salt and pepper to taste
1 tablespoon olive oil
Instructions
1. Heat the oil in a soup pot over medium heat. Add onion and garlic, sauté until softened.
2. Add the mushrooms to the pot and cook until they release their moisture.
3. Stir in millet, vegetable broth, thyme, and bay leaf. Bring to a boil.
4. Reduce heat, cover, and simmer for 20-25 minutes until millet is tender.
5. Remove bay leaf, season with salt and pepper, and serve hot.
Nutritional Info: Calories: 280, Protein: 9g, Carbohydrates: 50g, Fat: 5g, Fiber: 8g

Almond Flour Carrot Soup

A creamy and velvety soup made with sweet carrots and almond flour for added richness.
Preparation Time: 10 minutes
Cooking Time: 25 minutes
Total Time: 35 minutes
Servings: 4
Ingredients
4 large carrots, peeled and chopped
1 onion, diced
2 cloves garlic, minced
4 cups vegetable broth
1/4 cup almond flour
1 teaspoon ground cumin

Salt and pepper to taste
1 tablespoon olive oil

Instructions

1. Heat olive oil in a pot over medium heat.
2. Add onion and garlic, sauté until translucent.
3. Add chopped carrots and cook for a few minutes.
4. Sprinkle almond flour over the vegetables, stirring to coat evenly.
5. Pour in vegetable broth, add ground cumin, salt, and pepper. Bring to a boil.
6. Reduce heat, cover, and simmer for 20 minutes until carrots are tender.
7. Use an immersion blender or transfer to a blender to puree until smooth.
8. Adjust seasoning if needed and serve immediately. Enjoy!

Nutritional Info: Calories: 200, Protein: 5g, Carbohydrates: 25g, Fat: 10g, Fiber: 6g

Creamy Mushroom Quinoa Soup

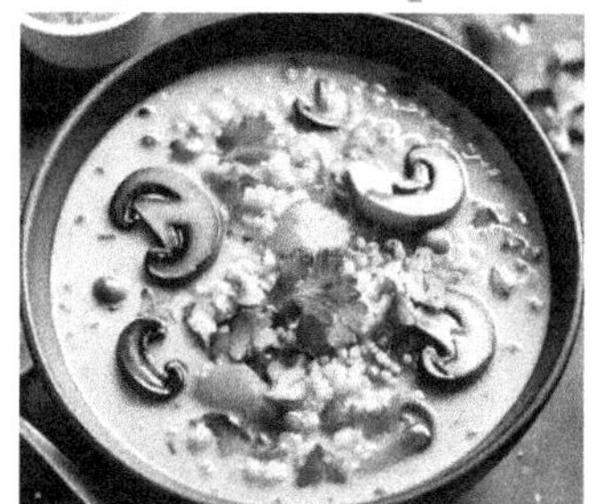

A creamy and satisfying soup featuring protein-packed quinoa and earthy mushrooms.

Preparation Time: 15 minutes
Cooking Time: 30 minutes
Total Time: 45 minutes
Servings: 4

Ingredients

1 cup quinoa, rinsed
4 cups vegetable broth
2 cups sliced mushrooms
1 onion, diced
2 cloves garlic, minced
1/2 cup coconut milk
1 tablespoon olive oil
1 teaspoon dried thyme
Salt and pepper to taste

Instructions

1. Heat olive oil in a pot over medium heat. Add onion and garlic, sauté until softened.
2. Add the mushrooms to the pot and cook until they release their moisture.
3. Stir in quinoa, vegetable broth, and thyme. Bring to a boil.
4. Reduce heat, cover, and simmer for 20-25 minutes until quinoa is cooked.
5. Stir in the milk and let it simmer for an additional 5 minutes.
6. Season with salt and pepper before serving.

Nutritional Info: Calories: 280, Protein: 9g, Carbohydrates: 35g, Fat: 10g, Fiber: 6g

Carrot Ginger Millet Soup

A vibrant and flavorful soup featuring the sweetness of carrots and the warmth of ginger.
Preparation Time: 10 minutes
Cooking Time: 25 minutes
Total Time: 35 minutes
Servings: 4
Ingredients
4 large carrots, peeled and chopped
1 onion, diced
2 cloves garlic, minced
1-inch piece of ginger, grated
1/2 cup millet, rinsed
4 cups vegetable broth
1 tablespoon olive oil
Salt and pepper to taste
Instructions
1. Heat olive oil in a pot over medium heat.
2. Add onion, garlic, and ginger, sauté until fragrant.
3. Add chopped carrots and cook for a few minutes.
4. Stir in millet and vegetable broth. Bring to a boil.
5. Reduce heat, cover, and simmer for 20 minutes until millet and carrots are tender.
6. Use an immersion blender or transfer to a blender to puree until smooth.
7. Season with salt and pepper before serving.
Nutritional Info: Calories: 230, Protein: 6g, Carbohydrates: 40g, Fat: 4g, Fiber: 8g

SALAD

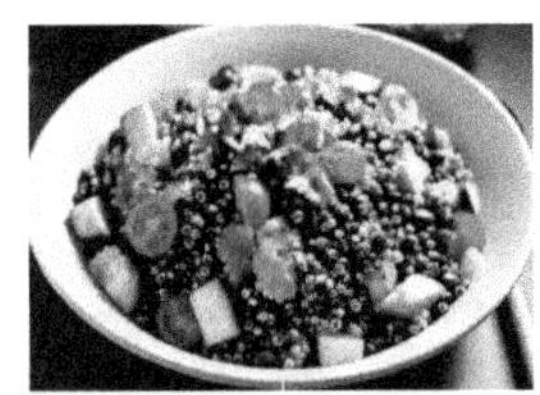

Quinoa and Black Bean Salad

A protein-packed salad featuring fluffy quinoa, black beans, and vibrant vegetables, tossed in a zesty lime dressing.
Preparation Time: 15 minutes
Total Time: 20 minutes
Servings: 4
Ingredients
1 cup cooked quinoa

1 can black beans (15 oz.) drained and rinsed
1 red bell pepper, diced
1 cup corn kernels
1/4 cup chopped cilantro
Juice of 2 limes
2 tablespoons olive oil
1 teaspoon cumin
Salt and pepper to taste
Instructions
1. In a large bowl, combine cooked quinoa, black beans, diced bell pepper, corn kernels, and chopped cilantro.
2. In a small bowl, whisk together lime juice, olive oil, cumin, salt, and pepper to make the dressing.
3. Pour the dressing over the salad and toss to combine.
4. Serve chilled.
Nutritional Info: Calories: 280, Protein: 10g, Carbohydrates: 40g, Fat: 8g, Fiber: 8g

Chickpea and Avocado Salad

Creamy avocado and protein-rich chickpeas are paired with crunchy vegetables and tangy lemon dressing in this refreshing salad.
Preparation Time: 10 minutes
Total Time: 10 minutes
Servings: 2
Ingredients
1 can (15 oz) chickpeas, drained and rinsed
1 avocado, diced
1 cucumber, diced
1/2 red onion, thinly sliced
Juice of 1 lemon
2 tablespoons olive oil
1 tablespoon chopped fresh parsley
Salt and pepper to taste
Instructions
1. In a large bowl, combine chickpeas, diced avocado, cucumber, and sliced red onion.
2. In a small bowl, whisk together lemon juice, olive oil, chopped parsley, salt, and pepper to make the dressing.
3. Pour the dressing over the salad and toss gently to coat.
4. Serve immediately.
Nutritional Info: Calories: 320, Protein: 10g, Carbohydrates: 30g, Fat: 18g, Fiber: 12g

Rainbow Kale Salad

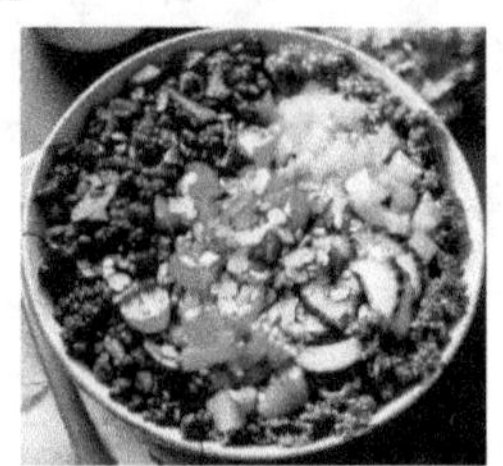

A colorful and nutrient-packed salad featuring kale, bell peppers, carrots, and cranberries, tossed in a tangy balsamic vinaigrette.

Preparation Time: 15 minutes

Total Time: 15 minutes

Servings: 4

Ingredients

4 cups chopped kale

1 red bell pepper, thinly sliced

1 yellow bell pepper, thinly sliced

1 carrot, grated

1/4 cup dried cranberries

1/4 cup sliced almonds

2 tablespoons balsamic vinegar

1 tablespoon maple syrup

1 tablespoon Dijon mustard

2 tablespoons olive oil

Salt and pepper to taste

Instructions

1. In a large bowl, massage chopped kale with a drizzle of olive oil until slightly softened.

2. Add sliced bell peppers, grated carrot, dried cranberries, and sliced almonds to the bowl.

3. In a small bowl, whisk together balsamic vinegar, maple syrup, Dijon mustard, olive oil, salt, and pepper to make the dressing.

4. Pour the dressing over the salad and toss to coat.

5. Serve immediately.

Nutritional Info: Calories: 240, Protein: 6g, Carbohydrates: 30g, Fat: 12g, Fiber: 6g

Apple, Carrot, and Almond Salad with Lemon Dressing

A vibrant salad bursting with flavors and textures.

Preparation Time: 15 minutes

Cooking Time: 0 minutes

Total Time: 15 minutes

Servings: 2

Ingredients

2 cups mixed greens

1 apple, thinly sliced

1 carrot, grated
1/4 cup sliced almonds
2 tablespoons lemon juice
1 tablespoon olive oil
1 teaspoon honey or maple syrup
Salt and pepper to taste
Instructions
1. In a large bowl, combine mixed greens, thinly sliced apple, grated carrot, and sliced almonds.
2. In a small bowl, whisk together lemon juice, olive oil, honey or maple syrup, salt, and pepper to make the dressing.
3. Drizzle the dressing over the salad and toss to coat evenly.
4. Serve immediately.
Nutritional Info: Calories: 220, Protein: 5g, Carbohydrates: 30g, Fat:10g, Fiber:8g

Mango and Black Bean Salad

Sweet mangoes, black beans, and colorful vegetables are tossed in a cilantro-lime dressing, creating a refreshing and satisfying salad.
Preparation Time: 15 minutes
Total Time: 15 minutes
Servings: 4
Ingredients
1 ripe mango, diced
1 can (15 oz) black beans, drained and rinsed
1 red bell pepper, diced
1/2 red onion, thinly sliced
1/4 cup chopped fresh cilantro
Juice of 2 limes
2 tablespoons olive oil
Salt and pepper to taste
Instructions
1. In a large bowl, combine diced mango, black beans, diced red bell pepper, thinly sliced red onion, and chopped cilantro.
2. In a small bowl, whisk together lime juice, olive oil, salt, and pepper to make the dressing.
3. Pour the dressing over the salad and toss gently to coat.
4. Serve chilled.
Nutritional Info: Calories: 280, Protein: 8g, Carbohydrates: 40g, Fat: 10g, Fiber: 10g

Greek Quinoa Salad

This Greek-inspired salad features protein-rich quinoa, cucumbers, tomatoes, olives, and tangy feta cheese, all tossed in a lemon-herb dressing.
Preparation Time: 15 minutes
Total Time: 20 minutes
Servings: 4
Ingredients

1 cup cooked quinoa
1 cucumber, diced
1 cup cherry tomatoes, halved
1/2 cup sliced Kalamata olives
1/4 cup crumbled feta cheese (optional)
Juice of 1 lemon
2 tablespoons olive oil
1 tablespoon chopped fresh parsley
1 teaspoon dried oregano
Salt and pepper to taste

Instructions

1. In a large bowl, combine cooked quinoa, diced cucumber, halved cherry tomatoes, sliced Kalamata olives, and crumbled feta cheese (if using).
2. In a small bowl, whisk together lemon juice, olive oil, chopped parsley, dried oregano, salt, and pepper to make the dressing.
3. Pour the dressing over the salad and toss gently to coat.
4. Serve chilled.

Nutritional Info: Calories: 280, Protein: 8g, Carbohydrates: 35g, Fat: 12g, Fiber: 6g

Roasted Beet and Arugula Salad

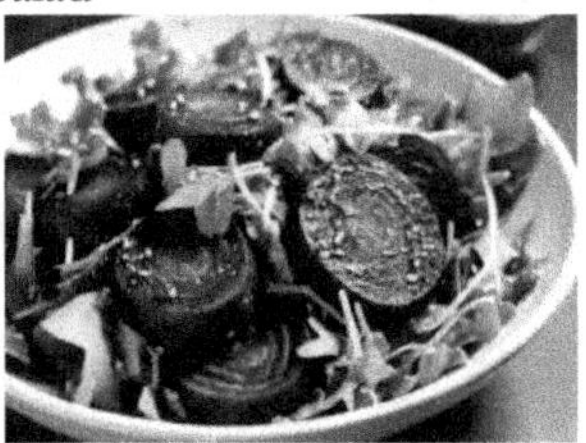

Earthy roasted beets are paired with peppery arugula, creamy avocado, and crunchy walnuts in this elegant salad.

Preparation Time: 15 minutes
Cooking Time: 45 minutes (for roasting beets)
Total Time: 1 hour
Servings: 2

Ingredients

2 medium beets, peeled and diced
4 cups arugula
1 avocado, diced
1/4 cup chopped walnuts
2 tablespoons balsamic vinegar
1 tablespoon olive oil
Salt and pepper to taste

Instructions

1. Preheat oven to 400°F (200°C).
2. Place diced beets on a baking sheet and drizzle with olive oil.
3. Season with salt and pepper.
4. Roast in the oven for 45 minutes or until beets are tender.
5. In a large bowl, combine arugula, diced avocado, chopped walnuts, and roasted beets.

6. Drizzle with balsamic vinegar and olive oil.
7. Toss gently to coat. Serve immediately.
Nutritional Info: Calories: 320, Protein: 6g, Carbohydrates: 20g, Fat: 22g, Fiber: 8g

Asian-Inspired Edamame Salad

This vibrant salad features protein-rich edamame, crunchy cabbage, carrots, and bell peppers, all tossed in a sesame ginger dressing.
Preparation Time: 15 minutes
Total Time: 15 minutes
Servings: 4
Ingredients
2 cups cooked edamame
2 cups shredded cabbage
1 carrot, grated
1 red bell pepper, thinly sliced
1/4 cup sliced green onions
2 tablespoons sesame seeds
2 tablespoons rice vinegar
1 tablespoon soy sauce or tamari
1 tablespoon sesame oil
1 teaspoon grated ginger
1 clove garlic, minced
1 teaspoon maple syrup
Salt and pepper to taste
Instructions
1. In a large bowl, combine cooked edamame, shredded cabbage, grated carrot, thinly sliced red bell pepper, sliced green onions, and sesame seeds.
2. In a small bowl, whisk together rice vinegar, soy sauce, sesame oil, grated ginger, minced garlic, maple syrup, salt, and pepper to make the dressing.
3. Pour the dressing over the salad and toss to coat.
4. Serve chilled.
Nutritional Info: Calories: 280, Protein: 14g, Carbohydrates: 25g, Fat: 14g, Fiber: 8

Summer Berry Spinach Salad

A refreshing salad featuring baby spinach, juicy berries, creamy avocado, and crunchy almonds, dressed in a tangy balsamic vinaigrette.
Preparation Time: 10 minutes
Total Time: 10 minutes
Servings: 2
Ingredients
4 cups baby spinach
1 cup mixed berries (e.g., strawberries, blueberries, raspberries)
1 avocado, diced
1/4 cup sliced almonds
2 tablespoons balsamic vinegar
1 tablespoon olive oil

1 teaspoon Dijon mustard
1 teaspoon maple syrup
Salt and pepper to taste
Instructions
1. In a large bowl, combine baby spinach, mixed berries, diced avocado, and sliced almonds.
2. In a small bowl, whisk together balsamic vinegar, olive oil, Dijon mustard, maple syrup, salt, and pepper to make the dressing.
3. Pour the dressing over the salad and toss gently to coat.
4. Serve immediately.
Nutritional Info: Calories: 280, Protein: 8g, Carbohydrates: 20g, Fat: 18g, Fiber: 8g

Tangy Cucumber and Tomato Salad

Crisp cucumbers and juicy tomatoes are tossed in a tangy lemon dill dressing, creating a refreshing and light salad.
Preparation Time: 10 minutes
Total Time: 10 minutes
Serving: 4
Ingredients
2 cucumbers, thinly sliced
2 cups cherry tomatoes, halved
1/4 cup chopped fresh dill
Juice of 1 lemon
2 tablespoons olive oil
Salt and pepper to taste
Instructions
1. In a large bowl, combine thinly sliced cucumbers, halved cherry tomatoes, and chopped fresh dill.
2. In a small bowl, whisk together lemon juice, olive oil, salt, and pepper to make the dressing.
3. Pour the dressing over the salad and toss gently to coat.
4. Serve chilled.
Nutritional Info: Calories: 120, Protein: 4g, Carbohydrates: 15g, Fat: 7g, Fiber: 5g

Southwest Quinoa Salad

A hearty salad featuring southwestern flavors with quinoa, black beans, corn, avocado, and a creamy cilantro lime dressing.
Preparation Time: 15 minutes
Total Time: 15 minutes
Serving Size: 4 servings
Ingredients:
1 cup cooked quinoa
1 can (15 oz) black beans, drained and rinsed
1 cup corn kernels
1 avocado, diced
1/4 cup chopped fresh cilantro

Juice of 2 limes
2 tablespoons olive oil
1 teaspoon cumin
Salt and pepper to taste

Instructions

1. In a large bowl, combine cooked quinoa, black beans, corn kernels, diced avocado, and chopped fresh cilantro.
2. In a small bowl, whisk together lime juice, olive oil, cumin, salt, and pepper to make the dressing.
3. Pour the dressing over the salad and toss gently to coat.
4. Serve chilled.

*Nutritional Info: Calories: 320, Protein: 10g, Carbohydrates: 40g, Fat: 14g, Fiber: 10g*Spiralized Zucchini Salad with Lemon-Herb Dressing

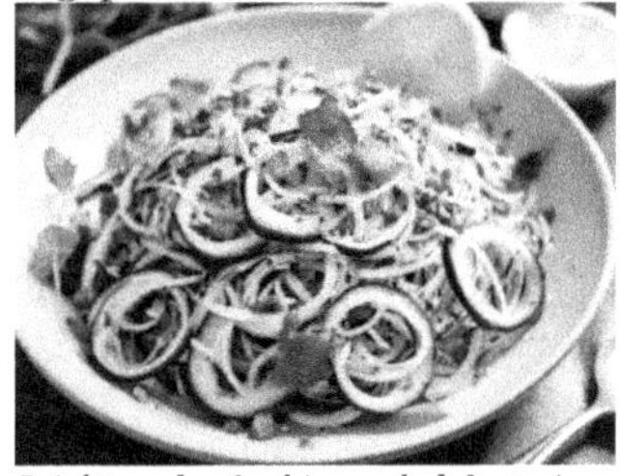

Light and refreshing salad featuring spiralized zucchini noodles tossed in a tangy lemon-herb dressing with cherry tomatoes and pine nuts.

Preparation Time: 15mins

Total Time: 15mins

Servings: 2

Ingredients:

2 medium zucchini, spiralized
1 cup cherry tomatoes, halved
2 tablespoons pine nuts
Juice of 1 lemon
2 tablespoons olive oil
1 tablespoon chopped fresh basil
1 tablespoon chopped fresh parsley
Salt and pepper to taste

Instructions

1. In a large bowl, combine spiralized zucchini noodles, halved cherry tomatoes, and pine nuts.
2. In a small bowl, whisk together lemon juice, olive oil, chopped fresh basil, chopped fresh parsley, salt, and pepper to make the dressing.
3. Pour the dressing over the salad and toss gently to coat.
4. Serve immediately.

Nutritional Info: Calories: 180, Protein: 5g, Carbohydrates: 15g, Fat: 12g, Fiber: 6g

Mediterranean Chickpea Salad

A vibrant and flavorful salad featuring chickpeas, cucumbers, tomatoes, olives, and feta cheese, dressed in a tangy Greek vinaigrette.

Preparation Time: 15mins

Total Time: 15mins

Serving: 4

Ingredients

1 can (15 oz) chickpeas, drained and rinsed

1 cucumber, diced

1 cup cherry tomatoes, halved

1/4 cup sliced Kalamata olives

1/4 cup crumbled feta cheese

2 tablespoons red wine vinegar

2 tablespoons olive oil

1 teaspoon dried oregano

Salt and pepper to taste

Instructions

1. In a large bowl, combine chickpeas, diced cucumber, halved cherry tomatoes, sliced Kalamata olives, and crumbled feta cheese.

2. In a small bowl, whisk together red wine vinegar, olive oil, dried oregano, salt, and pepper to make the dressing.

3. Pour the dressing over the salad and toss gently to coat.

4. Serve chilled.

Nutritional Info: Calories: 280, Protein: 10g, Carbohydrates: 25g, Fat: 16g, Fiber: 8g

Spinach and Strawberry Salad with Balsamic Dressing

A delightful combination of fresh baby spinach, juicy strawberries, creamy avocado, and crunchy almonds, drizzled with a tangy balsamic dressing.

Preparation Time: 10mins

Total Time: 10mins

Servings: 2

Ingredients

4 cups baby spinach

1 cup sliced strawberries

1 avocado, diced

1/4 cup sliced almonds

2 tablespoons balsamic vinegar

1 tablespoon olive oil

1 teaspoon Dijon mustard

1 teaspoon maple syrup

Salt and pepper to taste

Instructions

1. In a large bowl, combine baby spinach, sliced strawberries, diced avocado, and sliced almonds.

2. In a small bowl, whisk together balsamic vinegar, olive oil, Dijon mustard, maple syrup, salt, and pepper to make the dressing.

3. Pour the dressing over the salad and toss gently to coat.
4. Serve immediately.
Nutritional Info: Calories: 280, Protein: 8g, Carbohydrates: 20g, Fat: 18g, Fiber: 8g

Crispy Chickpea and Kale Caesar Salad

A hearty and satisfying salad featuring crispy roasted chickpeas, massaged kale, vegan Caesar dressing, and crunchy croutons.
Preparation Time: 15mins
Cooking Time: 30mins
Total Time: 45mins
Servings: 2
Ingredients
1 can (15 oz) chickpeas, drained and rinsed
4 cups chopped kale
2 tablespoons olive oil
Salt and pepper to taste
Vegan Caesar dressing (store-bought or homemade)
Vegan croutons
Instructions
1. Preheat oven to 400°F (200°C).
2. Pat dry chickpeas with a paper towel and place them on a baking sheet.
3. Drizzle with the oil, salt, and pepper.
4. Roast in the oven for 25-30 minutes until crispy.
5. In a large bowl, massage chopped kale with a drizzle of olive oil until slightly softened.
6. Add crispy chickpeas and vegan Caesar dressing to the bowl. Toss to coat.
7. Serve topped with vegan croutons.
Nutritional Info: Calories: 320, Protein: 10g, Carbohydrates: 25g, Fat: 18g, Fiber: 10g

Spring Asparagus and Radish Salad

A fresh and vibrant salad featuring tender asparagus spears, crisp radishes, peppery arugula, and a lemon dijon dressing.
Preparation Time: 10mins
Cooking Time: 5mins
Total Time: 15mins
Servings: 2
Ingredients
1 bunch asparagus, trimmed and halved
1 cup thinly sliced radishes
2 cups arugula
Juice of 1 lemon
2 tablespoons olive oil
1 teaspoon Dijon mustard
1 teaspoon maple syrup
Salt and pepper to taste
Instructions

1. Bring a pot of water to a boil.
2. Blanch asparagus spears in boiling water for 2-3 minutes until bright green and tender-crisp.
3. Immediately transfer to an ice bath to cool.
4. In a large bowl, combine blanched asparagus spears, thinly sliced radishes, and arugula.
5. In a small bowl, whisk together lemon juice, olive oil, Dijon mustard, maple syrup, salt, and pepper to make the dressing.
6. Pour the dressing over the salad and toss gently to coat.
7. Serve immediately.
Nutritional Info: Calories: 180, Protein: 6g, Carbohydrates: 15g, Fat: 12g, Fiber: 6g

Quinoa and Roasted Vegetable Salad

A hearty salad featuring fluffy quinoa, roasted vegetables, and a tangy lemon dressing.
Preparation Time: 15mins
Cooking Time: 25mins
Total Time: 40mins
Servings: 4

Ingredients
1 cup quinoa, rinsed
2 cups mixed vegetables (e.g., bell peppers, zucchini, eggplant), diced
2 tablespoons olive oil
Salt and pepper to taste
Juice of 1 lemon
2 tablespoons chopped fresh parsley
1/4 cup toasted pine nuts

Instructions
1. Preheat oven to 400°F (200°C).
2. In a medium saucepan, bring 2 cups of water to a boil.
3. Add quinoa, cover, and simmer for 15 minutes until fluffy.
4. Meanwhile, toss mixed vegetables with olive oil, salt, and pepper on a baking sheet.
5. Roast in the oven for 20-25 minutes until tender and lightly browned.
6. In a large bowl, combine cooked quinoa, roasted vegetables, lemon juice, chopped parsley, and toasted pine nuts. Toss gently to combine.
7. Serve warm or chilled.
Nutritional Info: Calories: 280, Protein: 8g, Carbohydrates: 35g, Fat: 12g, Fiber: 6g
Summer Berry and Spinach Salad with Almond Vinaigrette

A refreshing salad featuring baby spinach, ripe berries, crunchy almonds, and a sweet almond vinaigrette.
Preparation Time: 10mins
Total Time: 10mins
Servings: 2

Ingredients
4 cups baby spinach
1 cup mixed berries (e.g., strawberries, raspberries, blueberries,)

1/4 cup sliced almonds
2 tablespoons almond butter
2 tablespoons apple cider vinegar
1 tablespoon maple syrup
1 tablespoon water
Salt to taste

Instructions

1. In a large bowl, combine baby spinach, mixed berries, and sliced almonds.
2. In a small bowl, whisk together almond butter, apple cider vinegar, maple syrup, water, and salt to make the vinaigrette.
3. Pour the vinaigrette over the salad and toss gently to coat.
4. Serve immediately.

Nutritional Info: Calories: 220, Protein: 6g, Carbohydrates: 20g, Fat: 14g, Fiber: 8g

Mango and Black Bean Quinoa Salad

A tropical-inspired salad featuring sweet mangoes, protein-rich black beans, quinoa, and a zesty lime dressing.

Preparation Time: 15mins
Total Time: 15mins
Servings: 4

Ingredients

1 cup quinoa, rinsed
1 ripe mango, diced
1 can (15 oz) black beans, drained and rinsed
1/4 cup chopped fresh cilantro
Juice of 2 limes
2 tablespoons olive oil
Salt and pepper to taste

Instructions

1. In a medium saucepan, bring 2 cups of water to a boil.
2. Add quinoa, cover, and simmer for 15 minutes until fluffy.
3. In a large bowl, combine cooked quinoa, diced mango, black beans, chopped cilantro, lime juice, olive oil, salt, and pepper.
4. Toss gently to combine.
5. Serve chilled.

Nutritional Info: Calories: 320, Protein: 10g, Carbohydrates: 50g, Fat: 8g, Fiber: 12g

Asian-Inspired Forbidden Rice Salad

A colorful salad featuring forbidden rice, crunchy vegetables, and sesame ginger dressing.

Preparation Time: 20 minutes
Cooking Time: 30 minutes
Total Time: 50 minutes
Servings: 4

Ingredients

1 cup forbidden rice
2 cups water

1 cup shredded red cabbage
1 carrot, julienned
1 bell pepper, thinly sliced
1/4 cup sliced green onions
2 tablespoons sesame seeds
2 tablespoons rice vinegar
1 tablespoon tamari or soy sauce
1 tablespoon sesame oil
1 teaspoon grated ginger
1 clove garlic, minced
1 teaspoon maple syrup

Instructions

1. Rinse forbidden rice under cold water.
2. In a saucepan, combine rice and water.
3. Bring to a boil, then reduce heat to low, cover, and simmer for 30 minutes until rice is tender and water is absorbed.
4.In a large bowl, combine cooked forbidden rice, shredded red cabbage, julienned carrot, thinly sliced bell pepper, sliced green onions, and sesame seeds.
5. In a small bowl, whisk together rice vinegar, tamari, sesame oil, grated ginger, minced garlic, and maple syrup to make the dressing.
6. Pour the dressing over the salad and toss gently to coat.
7. Serve chilled.

Nutritional Info: Calories: 280, Protein: 6g, Carbohydrates: 45g, Fat: 8g, Fiber: 6g

Chickpea and Quinoa Greek Salad

A Mediterranean-inspired salad featuring chickpeas, quinoa, tomatoes, cucumbers, olives, and a lemon-herb dressing.

Preparation Time: 15mins
Cooking Time: 15mins
Total Time: 30mins
Serving: 4s

Ingredients

1 cup quinoa, rinsed
2 cups water
1 can (15 oz) chickpeas, drained and rinsed
1 cup cherry tomatoes, halved
1 cucumber, diced
1/4 cup sliced Kalamata olives
1/4 cup crumbled feta cheese (optional)
Juice of 1 lemon
2 tablespoons olive oil
1 tablespoon chopped fresh parsley
1 teaspoon dried oregano
Salt and pepper to taste

Instructions

1. In a saucepan, combine quinoa and water.

2. Bring to a boil, then reduce heat to low, cover, and simmer for 15 minutes until quinoa is fluffy and water is absorbed.
3. In a large bowl, combine cooked quinoa, chickpeas, halved cherry tomatoes, diced cucumber, sliced Kalamata olives, and crumbled feta cheese (if using).
4. In a small bowl, whisk together lemon juice, olive oil, chopped parsley, dried oregano, salt, and pepper to make the dressing.
5. Pour the dressing over the salad and toss gently to coat.
6. Serve chilled.
Nutritional Info: Calories: 320, Protein: 12g, Carbohydrates: 40g, Fat: 12g, Fiber: 8g

Rainbow Veggie Quinoa Salad with Lemon-Tahini Dressing

A vibrant salad featuring colorful vegetables, protein-rich quinoa, and a creamy lemon-tahini dressing.

Preparation Time: 20mins
Cooking Time: 15mins
Total Time: 35mins
Servings: 4

Ingredients

1 cup quinoa, rinsed
2 cups water
1 cup cherry tomatoes, halved
1 bell pepper, diced
1 cucumber, diced
1 carrot, shredded
1/4 cup chopped fresh parsley
1/4 cup toasted sunflower seeds
Juice of 1 lemon
2 tablespoons tahini
1 tablespoon olive oil
1 clove garlic, minced
Salt and pepper to taste

Instructions

1. In a saucepan, combine quinoa and water.
2. Bring to a boil, then reduce heat to low, cover, and simmer for 15 minutes until quinoa is fluffy and water is absorbed.
3. In a large bowl, combine cooked quinoa, halved cherry tomatoes, diced bell pepper, diced cucumber, shredded carrot, chopped parsley, and toasted sunflower seeds.
4. In a small bowl, whisk together lemon juice, tahini, olive oil, minced garlic, salt, and pepper to make the dressing.
3. Pour the dressing over the salad and toss gently to coat.
4. Serve chilled.
Nutritional Info: Calories: 320, Protein: 10g, Carbohydrates: 40g, Fat: 14g, Fiber: 8g

Pear and Walnut Spinach Salad with Balsamic Vinaigrette

A simple and elegant salad featuring fresh spinach, juicy pears, crunchy walnuts, and a tangy balsamic vinaigrette.
Preparation Time: 10mins
Total Time: 10mins
Servings: 2
Ingredients
4 cups baby spinach
1 ripe pear, thinly sliced
1/4 cup chopped walnuts
2 tablespoons balsamic vinegar
1 tablespoon olive oil
1 teaspoon Dijon mustard
1 teaspoon maple syrup
Salt and pepper to taste
Instructions
1. In a large bowl, combine baby spinach, thinly sliced pear, and chopped walnuts.
2. In a small bowl, whisk together balsamic vinegar, olive oil, Dijon mustard, maple syrup, salt, and pepper to make the dressing.
3. Pour the dressing over the salad and toss gently to coat.
4. Serve immediately.
Nutritional Info: Calories: 240, Protein: 6g, Carbohydrates: 20g, Fat: 16g, Fiber: 8g

Zucchini Noodle Salad with Avocado Pesto

A light and refreshing salad featuring zucchini noodles tossed in creamy avocado pesto.
Preparation Time: 15mins
Total Time: 15mins
Servings: 2
Ingredients
2 medium zucchini, spiralized
1 ripe avocado
1 cup fresh basil leaves
1/4 cup pine nuts
Juice of 1 lemon
1 clove garlic
2 tablespoons olive oil
Salt and pepper to taste
Instructions
1. In a large bowl, toss spiralized zucchini noodles with a pinch of salt and let sit for 5 minutes to soften slightly.
2. Meanwhile, in a food processor, combine ripe avocado, basil leaves, pine nuts, lemon juice, garlic, olive oil, salt, and pepper.
3. Blend until smooth and creamy.
4. Pour the avocado pesto over the zucchini noodles and toss gently to coat.

5. Serve immediately.
Nutritional Info: Calories: 280, Protein: 6g, Carbohydrates: 15g, Fat: 22g, Fiber: 8g

Kale and Quinoa Salad with Cranberries and Almonds

A nutritious salad featuring massaged kale, protein-rich quinoa, sweet cranberries, and crunchy almonds, tossed in a tangy vinaigrette.

Preparation Time: 15mins
Cooking Time: 15mins
Total Time: 30mins
Servings: 4

Ingredients

1 cup quinoa, rinsed
2 cups water
4 cups chopped kale
1/4 cup dried cranberries
1/4 cup sliced almonds
Juice of 1 lemon
2 tablespoons olive oil
1 teaspoon Dijon mustard
1 teaspoon maple syrup
Salt and pepper to taste

Instructions

1. In a saucepan, combine quinoa and water.
2. Bring to a boil, then reduce heat to low, cover, and simmer for 15 minutes until quinoa is fluffy and water is absorbed.
3. In a large bowl, massage chopped kale with a drizzle of olive oil until slightly softened.
4. Add cooked quinoa, dried cranberries, sliced almonds, lemon juice, Dijon mustard, maple syrup, salt, and pepper to the bowl.
5. Toss gently to combine.
6. Serve chilled.
Nutritional Info: Calories: 280, Protein: 8g, Carbohydrates: 35g, Fat: 12g, Fiber: 6g

Warm Brussels Sprout and Sweet Potato Salad with Maple-Dijon Dressing

A cozy salad featuring roasted Brussels sprouts and sweet potatoes, tossed in a sweet and tangy maple-Dijon dressing.

Preparation Time: 15 minutes
Cooking Time: 30 minutes
Total Time: 45 minutes
Servings: 4

Ingredients

1 lb Brussels sprouts, trimmed and halved
1 large sweet potato, peeled and diced
2 tablespoons olive oil

Salt and pepper to taste
2 tablespoons maple syrup
1 tablespoon Dijon mustard
1 tablespoon apple cider vinegar
1/4 cup chopped pecans
Instructions
1. Preheat oven to 400°F (200°C).
2. On a baking sheet, toss Brussels sprouts and sweet potatoes with olive oil, salt, and pepper.
3. Roast in the oven for 25-30 minutes until tender and caramelized.
4. In a small bowl, whisk together maple syrup, Dijon mustard, and apple cider vinegar to make the dressing.
5. In a large bowl, combine roasted Brussels sprouts and sweet potatoes with chopped pecans.
6. Drizzle the dressing over the salad and toss gently to coat.
7. Serve warm.
Nutritional Info: Calories: 280, Protein: 6g, Carbohydrates: 35g, Fat: 14g, Fiber: 8g

SNACKS

Millet Energy Balls

These energy balls are packed with the goodness of millet and nuts, perfect for a quick snack on the go.
Preparation Time: 15 minutes
Cooking Time: 0 minutes
Total Time: 15 minutes
Servings: 12 balls
Ingredients
1 cup cooked millet
1/2 cup almond flour
1/4 cup maple syrup
1/4 cup almond butter
1/4 cup chopped walnuts
1/4 cup dried fruits (such as raisins or apricots), chopped
1 teaspoon vanilla extract
Instructions
1. In a mixing bowl, combine all ingredients until well combined.
2. Roll the mixture into small balls and place them on a baking sheet.
3. Refrigerate for at least 30 minutes before serving.
Nutritional Info: Calories: 120, Protein: 3g, Carbohydrates: 15g, Fat: 6g, Fiber: 2g

Quinoa and Vegetable Stuffed Peppers

These colorful stuffed peppers are filled with quinoa and vegetables, making them a satisfying and nutritious snack.

Preparation Time: 20 minutes
Cooking Time: 40 minutes
Total Time: 60 minutes
Servings: 4

Ingredients

4 large bell peppers, halved and seeds removed
1 cup cooked quinoa
1 cup diced carrots
1 cup diced zucchini
1/2 cup diced onion
1/2 cup diced tomatoes
2 cloves garlic, minced
1 teaspoon dried thyme
Salt and pepper to taste
2 tablespoons olive oil

Instructions

1. Preheat the oven to 375°F (190°C) and line a baking dish with parchment paper.
2. In a medium skillet, heat the oil over medium heat. Add onions and garlic in a heated oil, sauté until translucent.
3. Add carrots, zucchini, tomatoes, and dried thyme. Cook until vegetables are tender.
4. Stir in cooked quinoa and season with salt and pepper.
5. Stuff each pepper half with the quinoa and vegetable mixture.
6. Place stuffed peppers in the baking dish and cover with foil.
7. Bake for 30 minutes, then remove foil and bake for an additional 10 minutes.

Nutritional Info: Calories: 180, Protein: 5g, Carbohydrates: 25g, Fat: 6g, Fiber: 5g

Almond Flour Banana Muffins

These moist and fluffy muffins are made with almond flour and ripe bananas, perfect for a sweet and satisfying snack.

Preparation Time: 10 minutes
Cooking Time: 20 minutes
Total Time: 30 minutes
Servings: Makes 12 muffins

Ingredients

2 cups almond flour
3 ripe bananas, mashed
1/4 cup maple syrup
2 tablespoons coconut oil, melted
2 teaspoons baking powder
1 teaspoon vanilla extract
1/2 teaspoon cinnamon
Pinch of salt

Instructions

1. Preheat the oven to 350°F and properly line a muffin tin with paper liners.

2. In a large mixing bowl, combine almond flour, coconut oil, mashed bananas, maple syrup, baking powder, cinnamon, vanilla extract, and salt until well combined.
3. Divide the batter evenly among the muffin cups.
4. Bake for 18-20 minutes, until golden brown and a toothpick inserted into the center comes out clean.
5. Allow muffins to cool before serving.
Nutritional Info: Calories: 160, Protein: 4g, Carbohydrates: 15g, Fat: 10g, Fiber: 3g

Millet Energy Bars

These energy bars are packed with protein and fiber from millet and nuts, making them a nutritious and filling snack.
Preparation Time: 15 minutes
Cooking Time: 25 minutes
Total Time: 40 minutes
Servings: Makes 8 bars
Ingredients
1 cup cooked millet
1/2 cup almond flour
1/4 cup maple syrup
1/4 cup almond butter
1/4 cup chopped walnuts
1/4 cup dried fruits (such as cranberries or raisins)
1 teaspoon vanilla extract
Instructions
1. Preheat the oven to 350°F (175°C) and line a baking dish with parchment paper.
2. In a mixing bowl, combine all ingredients until well mixed.
3. Press the mixture into the prepared baking dish, smoothing the top with a spatula.
4. Bake for 25 minutes, or until lightly golden brown.
5. Remove from the heat let cool completely before cutting into bars.
Nutritional Info: Calories: 220, Protein: 6g, Carbohydrates: 25g, Fat: 11g, Fiber: 3g

Quinoa Salad Stuffed Avocado

This refreshing snack features quinoa salad stuffed into creamy avocado halves, perfect for a light and satisfying treat.
Preparation Time: 15 minutes
Cooking Time: 15 minutes
Total Time: 30 minutes
Servings: 4
Ingredients
2 avocados, halved and pitted
1 cup cooked quinoa
1/2 cup diced carrots
1/2 cup diced cucumber
1/4 cup diced red onion

1/4 cup chopped fresh parsley
2 tablespoons lemon juice
2 tablespoons olive oil
Salt and pepper to taste
Instructions
1. In a mixing bowl, combine cooked quinoa, carrots, cucumber, red onion, parsley, lemon juice, olive oil, salt, and pepper.
2. Spoon the quinoa salad into the avocado halves.
3. Serve immediately, or chill in the refrigerator until ready to serve.
Nutritional Info: Calories: 180, Protein: 4g, Carbohydrates: 15g, Fat: 12g, Fiber: 6g

Almond Flour Apple Muffins

These moist and flavorful muffins are made with almond flour and fresh apples, perfect for a wholesome and delicious snack.

Preparation Time: 15 minutes
Cooking Time: 25 minutes
Total Time: 40 minutes
Servings: 12 muffins
Ingredients
2 cups almond flour
1 teaspoon baking powder
1/2 teaspoon baking soda
1/4 teaspoon salt
1 teaspoon ground cinnamon
2 flax eggs (2 tablespoons ground flaxseed meal + 6 tablespoons water)
1/4 cup maple syrup
1/4 cup almond milk
1 teaspoon vanilla extract
1 cup grated apple (1 large apple will be fine)
Instructions
1. Preheat the oven to 350°F (175°C) and line a muffin tin with paper liners.
2. in a large mixing bowl, whisk together almond flour, baking powder, baking soda, salt, and cinnamon.
3. In a separate bowl, prepare the flax eggs by mixing ground flaxseed meal with water. Let sit for 5 minutes to thicken.
4. Stir maple syrup, almond milk, vanilla extract, and grated apple into the flax eggs.
5. Add the wet ingredients to the dry ingredients and stir well until just combined.
6. Divide the batter equally among the muffin cups.
7. Bake for about 23 minutes, or until a toothpick inserted into the center comes out clean.
8. Let cool before serving.
Nutritional Info: Calories: 180, Protein: 5g, Carbohydrates: 15g, Fat: 12g, Fiber: 3g

Carrot and Walnut Energy Bites

These bite-sized energy bites are packed with carrots, walnuts, and dates, providing a natural sweetness and crunch.

Preparation Time: 15 minutes
Cooking Time: 0 minutes
Total Time: 15 minutes
Servings: 12 bites

Ingredients

1 cup shredded carrots

1 cup walnuts

1 cup pitted dates

1/4 cup shredded coconut

1 teaspoon ground cinnamon

Pinch of salt

Instructions

1. in a food processor, pulse walnuts until finely chopped.
2. Add shredded carrots, dates, shredded coconut, cinnamon, and salt to the food processor.
3. Pulse until the mixture comes together and forms a sticky dough.
4. Roll the dough into small balls and place properly on a baking sheet lined with parchment paper.
5. Refrigerate for at least 30 minutes or more before serving.

Nutritional Info: Calories: 160, Protein: 3g, Carbohydrates: 20g, Fat: 8g, Fiber: 4g

Apple and Almond Butter Rice Cakes

These rice cakes topped with almond butter and sliced apples are a simple yet satisfying snack that provides a perfect balance of sweetness and crunch.

Preparation Time: 5 minutes
Cooking Time: 0 minutes
Total Time: 5 minutes
Servings: 2

Ingredients

2 rice cakes (gluten-free)

2 tablespoons almond butter

1 small apple, thinly sliced

Cinnamon for sprinkling (optional)

Instructions

1. Spread almond butter evenly onto each rice cake.
2. Top with sliced apples.
3. Sprinkle with cinnamon, if desired.
4. Serve immediately.

Nutritional Info: Calories: 200, Protein: 5g, Carbohydrates: 25g, Fat: 10g, Fiber: 4g

Carrot Cake Oatmeal Cookies

These soft and chewy oatmeal cookies are infused with the flavors of carrot cake, making them a delightful and wholesome snack.

Preparation Time: 15 minutes
Cooking Time: 12 minutes
Total Time: 27 minutes

Servings: 12 cookies
Ingredients
1 cup rolled oats (gluten-free)
1/2 cup almond flour
1/2 cup shredded carrots
1/4 cup chopped walnuts
1/4 cup raisins
1/4 cup maple syrup
1/4 cup coconut oil, melted
1 teaspoon ground cinnamon
1/2 teaspoon ground ginger
1/4 teaspoon ground nutmeg
Pinch of salt
Instructions
1. Preheat the oven to 350°F (175°C) and line a baking sheet with parchment paper.
2. In a mixing bowl, combine rolled oats, almond flour, shredded carrots, chopped walnuts, raisins, maple syrup, coconut oil, cinnamon, ginger, nutmeg, and salt.
3. Stir until all ingredients are well combined.
4. Drop spoonful's of dough onto the prepared baking sheet and flatten slightly with the back of a spoon.
5. Bake for 10-12 minutes, or until edges are golden brown.
6. Remove from the oven, let cool on the baking sheet for about 5 minutes before transferring to a wire rack to cool completely.
Nutritional Info: Calories: 180, Protein: 4g, Carbohydrates: 20g, Fat: 10g, Fiber: 3g

Apple Walnut Salad

This refreshing salad combines crisp apples, crunchy walnuts, and leafy greens for a satisfying and nutritious snack or side dish.
Preparation Time: 10 minutes
Cooking Time: 0 minutes
Total Time: 10 minutes
Servings: 2
Ingredients
2 cups mixed greens (such as arugula, spinach or kale)
1 apple, thinly sliced
1/4 cup chopped walnuts
2 tablespoons balsamic vinaigrette dressing
Instructions
1. In a large mixing bowl, toss mixed greens with sliced apples and chopped walnuts.
2. Drizzle with balsamic vinaigrette dressing and toss until evenly coated.
3. Divide the salad between two plates and serve immediately.
Nutritional Info: Calories: 200, Protein: 3g, Carbohydrates: 20g, Fat: 12g, Fiber: 5g

Fruit and Nut Trail Mix

This homemade trail mix is made with a variety of dried fruits and nuts, providing a tasty and convenient snack for any time of day.
Preparation Time: 5 minutes
Cooking Time: 0 minutes
Total Time: 5 minutes
Servings: 4
Ingredients
1/2 cup dried apricots, chopped
1/2 cup dried cranberries
1/2 cup dried cherries
1/2 cup raw almonds
1/2 cup raw cashews
1/2 cup pumpkin seeds
1/4 cup dark chocolate chips (optional)
Instructions
1. In a mixing bowl, combine all ingredients and toss until evenly distributed.
2. Divide the trail mix into individual servings or store in an airtight container for later use.
Nutritional Info: Calories: 220, Protein: 6g, Carbohydrates: 25g, Fat: 12g, Fiber: 4g

Baked Apple Chips

These crispy apple chips are a healthy alternative to store-bought snacks, and they're perfect for satisfying your crunchy cravings.
Preparation Time: 10 minutes
Cooking Time: 2 hours
Total Time: 2 hours 10 minutes
Servings: 4
Ingredients
2 apples, cored and thinly sliced
1 tablespoon lemon juice
1 teaspoon ground cinnamon
Instructions
1. Preheat the oven to 200°F and line a baking sheet with parchment paper.
2. In a large mixing bowl, toss apple slices with lemon juice and ground cinnamon until evenly coated.
3. Arrange the apple slices in a single layer on the prepared baking sheet.
4. Bake for 1 hour, then flip the apple slices and bake for an additional 1 hour, or until crispy.
5. Let cool completely before serving.
Nutritional Info: Calories: 80, Protein: 1g, Carbohydrates: 20g, Fat: 0g, Fiber: 4g

Quinoa Avocado Salad Bites

These bite-sized snacks are packed with protein and healthy fats, featuring creamy avocado and protein-rich quinoa.

Preparation Time: 15 minutes
Cooking Time: 15 minutes
Total Time: 30 minutes
Servings: Makes 12 bites

Ingredients

1 cup cooked quinoa
1 ripe avocado, mashed
2 tablespoons chopped cherry tomatoes
1 tablespoon chopped cilantro
1 tablespoon lime juice
Salt and pepper to taste

Instructions

1. In a bowl, mix together cooked quinoa, mashed avocado, cherry tomatoes, cilantro, lime juice, salt, and pepper.
2. Using a spoon, scoop the mixture onto small lettuce leaves or cucumber slices to create bite-sized servings.

Nutritional Info: Calories: 60, Protein: 2g, Carbohydrates: 6g, Fat: 3g, Fiber: 2g

Sweet Potato Hummus with Veggie Sticks

Creamy sweet potato hummus paired with fresh veggie sticks makes for a satisfying and nutritious snack.

Preparation Time: 10 minutes
Cooking Time: 25 minutes
Total Time: 35 minutes
Servings: 4

Ingredients

1 large sweet potato, peeled and diced
1 can (15 oz.) chickpeas, drained and rinsed
2 cloves garlic, minced
2 tablespoons tahini
2 tablespoons lemon juice
1 teaspoon ground cumin
Salt and pepper to taste
Assorted veggie sticks (carrots, cucumber, bell peppers) for serving

Instructions

1. Preheat oven to 400°F (200°C).
2. Roast diced sweet potato for 20-25 minutes until tender.
3. In a food processor, combine roasted sweet potato, chickpeas, garlic, tahini, lemon juice, cumin, salt, and pepper. Blend until smooth.
4. Serve the sweet potato hummus with assorted veggie sticks.

Nutritional Info: Calories: 160, Protein: 5g, Carbohydrates: 25g, Fat: 5g, Fiber: 6g

Crispy Baked Chickpeas

These crunchy chickpeas are seasoned to perfection, making them an addictive and protein-packed snack.

Preparation Time: 5 minutes

Cooking Time: 35 minutes
Total Time: 40 minutes
Servings: 4
Ingredients
2 cans chickpeas, (15 oz. each) drained and rinsed
2 tablespoons olive oil
1 teaspoon paprika
1/2 teaspoon garlic powder
1/2 teaspoon cumin
Salt and pepper to taste
Instructions
1. Preheat oven to 400°F (200°C). Line a baking sheet with parchment paper.
2. Pat dry the chickpeas with a paper towel to remove excess moisture.
4. In a bowl, toss chickpeas with olive oil, paprika, garlic powder, cumin, salt, and pepper.
5. Spread the seasoned chickpeas in a single layer on a prepared baking sheet.
6. Bake for 30-35 minutes until crispy, shaking the pan halfway through.
Nutritional Info: Calories: 210, Protein: 9g, Carbohydrates: 28g, Fat: 7g, Fiber: 8g

Zucchini Pizza Bites

These zucchini pizza bites are a delicious gluten-free alternative to traditional pizza, featuring zucchini slices topped with marinara sauce and dairy-free cheese.
Preparation Time: 10 minutes
Cooking Time: 15 minutes
Total Time: 25 minutes
Servings: 12 bites
Ingredients
2 medium zucchinis, sliced into rounds
1/2 cup marinara sauce
1/2 cup dairy-free cheese shreds
1 teaspoon dried oregano
1/2 teaspoon garlic powder
Salt and pepper to taste
Instructions
1. Preheat oven to 400°F (200°C).
2. Line a baking sheet with parchment paper.
3. Place zucchini rounds on the prepared baking sheet.
4. Top each round with marinara sauce, dairy-free cheese shreds, dried oregano, garlic powder, salt, and pepper.
5. Bake for 12-15 minutes until zucchini is tender and cheese is melted.
Nutritional Info: Calories: 35, Protein: 2g, Carbohydrates: 5g, Fat: 1g, Fiber: 1g

Fruit and Nut Energy Bites

These energy bites are packed with dried fruits, nuts, and seeds, providing a nutritious boost of energy.
Preparation Time: 10 minutes

Cooking Time: 0 minutes
Total Time: 10 minutes
Servings: 12 bites
Ingredients
1 cup Medjool dates, pitted
1/2 cup almonds
1/4 cup dried cranberries
1/4 cup shredded coconut
2 tablespoons chia seeds
1 tablespoon maple syrup
Instructions
1. In a food processor, combine pitted dates, almonds, dried cranberries, shredded coconut, chia seeds, and maple syrup.
2. Pulse until mixture comes together and forms a sticky dough.
3. Roll the dough into small balls, about 1 inch in diameter.
4. Store in an airtight container in the refrigerator until ready to eat.
Nutritional Info: Calories: 100, Protein: 2g, Carbohydrates: 15g, Fat: 4g, Fiber: 3g

Cucumber Avocado Rolls

These refreshing rolls feature thinly sliced cucumber filled with creamy avocado and crunchy vegetables, perfect for a light and healthy snack.
Preparation Time: 15 minutes
Cooking Time: 0 minutes
Total Time: 15 minutes
Servings: 8 rolls
Ingredients
1 large cucumber
1 ripe avocado, mashed
1/2 red bell pepper, thinly sliced
1/2 carrot, julienned
1/4 cup alfalfa sprouts
1 tablespoon lemon juice
Salt and pepper to taste
Instructions
1. Using a mandoline or vegetable peeler, slice the cucumber lengthwise into thin strips.
2. Spread mashed avocado onto each cucumber strip.
3. Top with sliced bell pepper, julienned carrot, alfalfa sprouts, lemon juice, salt, and pepper.
4. Roll up the cucumber strips and secure with toothpicks if necessary.
Nutritional Info: Calories: 40, Protein: 1g, Carbohydrates: 4g, Fat: 3g, Fiber: 2g

Quinoa Energy Bites

These energy bites are packed with protein and fiber, making them the perfect snack for a quick energy boost.
Preparation Time: 15 minutes

Cooking Time: 0 minutes
Total Time: 15 minutes
Servings: 12 energy bites

Ingredients

1 cup cooked quinoa
1/2 cup almond butter
1/4 cup maple syrup
1/4 cup shredded coconut
1/4 cup chopped nuts (such as walnuts or almonds)
1 teaspoon vanilla extract
Pinch of salt

Instructions

1. In a medium mixing bowl, combine all the ingredients.
2. Roll the mixture into small balls and place them on a baking sheet.
3. Refrigerate for at least 30 minutes before serving.

Nutritional Info: Calories: 120, Protein: 3g, Carbohydrates: 12g, Fat: 7g, Fiber: 2g

Chickpea Flour Pancakes

These savory pancakes are perfect for a quick and filling snack.
Preparation Time: 10 minutes
Cooking Time: 10 minutes
Total Time: 20 minutes
Servings: 4 pancakes

Ingredients

1 cup chickpea flour
1 cup water
1/4 teaspoon salt
1/4 teaspoon black pepper
1/4 teaspoon cumin
1/4 teaspoon paprika
1/4 cup chopped fresh herbs (such as parsley or cilantro)
1 tablespoon olive oil (for cooking)

Instructions

1. In a mixing bowl, whisk together chickpea flour, water, salt, pepper, cumin, paprika, and chopped herbs until smooth.
2. Heat the oil in a non-stick skillet over medium heat.
3. Pour 1/4 cup of batter into the skillet and spread it into a thin pancake.
4. Cook for 2-3 minutes on each side, until golden brown.
5. Repeat with the remaining batter.

Nutritional Info: Calories: 110, Protein: 5g, Carbohydrates: 14g, Fat: 4g, Fiber: 3g

Stuffed Mini Bell Peppers

These stuffed peppers are colorful, flavorful, and perfect for snacking.
Preparation Time: 15 minutes
Cooking Time: 15 minutes
Total Time: 30 minutes

Servings: 12 stuffed peppers

Ingredients

12 mini bell peppers, halved and seeds removed

1 cup cooked quinoa

1/2 cup black beans, drained and rinsed

1/2 cup corn kernels (fresh or frozen)

1/4 cup diced tomatoes

1/4 cup chopped fresh cilantro

1 teaspoon chili powder

1/2 teaspoon cumin

Salt and pepper to taste

Instructions

1. Preheat the oven to 375°F and line a baking sheet with parchment paper.

2. In a mixing bowl, combine quinoa, black beans, corn, tomatoes, cilantro, chili powder, cumin, salt, and pepper.

3. Spoon the quinoa mixture into each pepper half and place them on the prepared baking sheet.

4. Bake for 15 minutes, until the peppers are tender.

Nutritional Info: Calories: 60, Protein: 2g, Carbohydrates: 12g, Fat: 1g, Fiber: 2g

Crispy Baked Kale Chips

These crunchy kale chips are a healthy alternative to potato chips.

Preparation Time: 10 minutes

Cooking Time: 15 minutes

Total Time: 25 minutes

Servings: 4

Ingredients

1 bunch kale, washed and dried

1 tablespoon olive oil

1 tablespoon nutritional yeast

1/2 teaspoon garlic powder

Salt to taste

Instructions

1. Preheat the oven to 300°F (150°C) and line a baking sheet with parchment paper.

2. Remove the stems from the kale leaves and tear them into bite-sized pieces.

3. In a large bowl, massage kale leaves with olive oil, nutritional yeast, garlic powder, and salt until evenly coated.

4. Spread the kale leaves in a single layer on the prepared baking sheet.

5. Bake for 10-15 minutes, until crispy.

Nutritional Info: Calories: 50, Protein: 2g, Carbohydrates: 5g, Fat: 3g, Fiber: 2g

Sweet Potato Hummus

This creamy hummus is made with sweet potatoes for a unique twist on a classic snack.

Preparation Time: 10 minutes

Cooking Time: 40 minutes

Total Time: 50 minutes
Servings: 2 cups
Ingredients
2 medium sweet potatoes, peeled and diced
1 can (15 ounces) chickpeas, drained and rinsed
2 cloves garlic, minced
1/4 cup tahini
1/4 cup lemon juice
2 tablespoons olive oil
1 teaspoon cumin
Salt and pepper to taste
Instructions
1. Preheat the oven to 400°F and line a baking sheet with parchment paper.
2. Place diced sweet potatoes on the prepared baking sheet and roast for 30-40 minutes, until tender.
3. In a food processor, combine roasted sweet potatoes, chickpeas, garlic, tahini, lemon juice, olive oil, cumin, salt, and pepper.
4. Blend until smooth, adding water as needed to reach desired consistency.
5. Serve with sliced vegetables or gluten-free crackers.
Nutritional Info: Calories: 120, Protein: 4g, Carbohydrates: 14g, Fat: 6g, Fiber: 3g

Rice Paper Spring Rolls

These fresh and colorful spring rolls are filled with crisp vegetables and served with a tangy dipping sauce.
Preparation Time: 20 minutes
Cooking Time: 0 minutes
Total Time: 20 minutes
Servings: 8 spring rolls
Ingredients
8 rice paper wrappers
2 cups shredded lettuce
1 cup matchstick carrots
1 cup thinly sliced cucumber
1/2 cup sliced bell peppers
1/2 cup fresh mint leaves
1/2 cup fresh cilantro leaves
1/4 cup chopped peanuts (optional)
Instructions
1. Fill a shallow dish with warm water.
2. Dip one rice paper wrapper into the water for a few seconds until softened.
3. Place the softened wrapper on a clean surface and add a small handful of lettuce, carrots, cucumber, bell peppers, mint, cilantro, and chopped peanuts (if using) in the center.
4. Fold the bottom of the wrapper over the filling, then fold in the sides, and roll tightly.
5. Repeat with the remaining wrappers and filling ingredients.

6. Serve with your favorite dipping sauce, such as peanut or hoisin sauce.
Nutritional Info: Calories: 70, Protein: 2g, Carbohydrates: 15g, Fat: 1g, Fiber: 2g

Cauliflower Buffalo Wings

These crispy cauliflower wings are coated in spicy buffalo sauce for a delicious and healthy snack.
Preparation Time: 15 minutes
Cooking Time: 25 minutes
Total Time: 40 minutes
Servings: 4
Ingredients
1 head cauliflower, cut into florets
1/2 cup gluten-free flour
1/2 cup water
1 teaspoon garlic powder
1/2 teaspoon paprika
Salt and pepper to taste
1/2 cup hot sauce
2 tablespoons melted vegan butter
Instructions
1. Preheat the oven to 450°F (230°C) and line a baking sheet with parchment paper.
2. In a large bowl, whisk together gluten-free flour, water, garlic powder, paprika, salt, and pepper until smooth.
3. Dip cauliflower florets into the batter, shaking off any excess, and place them on the prepared baking sheet.
4. Bake for 20 minutes, flipping halfway through, until cauliflower is golden brown and crispy.
5. In a separate bowl, combine hot sauce and melted vegan butter.
6. Place the baked cauliflower in the buffalo sauce and toss well to coat evenly
7. Return cauliflower to the baking sheet and bake for an additional 5 minutes.
Nutritional Info: Calories: 110, Protein: 3g, Carbohydrates: 15g, Fat: 4g, Fiber: 3g

Almond Butter Banana Sushi

This fun twist on sushi features bananas and almond butter rolled in a gluten-free tortilla.
Preparation Time: 10 minutes
Cooking Time: 0 minutes
Total Time: 10 minutes
Servings: 4 rolls
Ingredients
2 large gluten-free tortillas
1/2 cup almond butter
2 bananas
2 tablespoons chia seeds
2 tablespoons shredded coconut
Instructions
1. Lay out a tortilla and spread a layer of almond butter over the entire surface.

2. Place a banana along one edge of the tortilla and sprinkle with chia seeds and shredded coconut.
3. Roll the tortilla tightly around the banana, pressing gently to seal.
4. Repeat with the remaining tortilla and ingredients.
5. Slice each roll into bite-sized pieces and serve.
Nutritional Info: Calories: 180, Protein: 5g, Carbohydrates: 20g, Fat: 10g, Fiber: 5g

Roasted Chickpeas

These crunchy roasted chickpeas are seasoned with spices for a flavorful and satisfying snack.
Preparation Time: 5 minutes
Cooking Time: 35 minutes
Total Time: 40 minutes
Servings: 4
Ingredients
2 cans (15 ounces each) chickpeas, drained and rinsed
2 tablespoons olive oil
1 teaspoon cumin
1 teaspoon paprika
1/2 teaspoon garlic powder
Salt and pepper to taste
Instructions
1. Preheat the oven to 400°F (200°C) and line a baking sheet with parchment paper.
2. Pat chickpeas dry with a clean kitchen towel or paper towels to remove excess moisture.
3. In a mixing bowl, toss chickpeas with olive oil, cumin, paprika, garlic powder, salt, and pepper until evenly coated.
4. Spread chickpeas in a single layer on the prepared baking sheet.
5. Bake for 30-35 minutes, stirring halfway through, until chickpeas are golden and crispy.
6. Allow chickpeas to cool slightly before serving.
Nutritional Info: Calories: 150, Protein: 6g, Carbohydrates: 18g, Fat: 6g, Fiber: 5g

DESSERTS

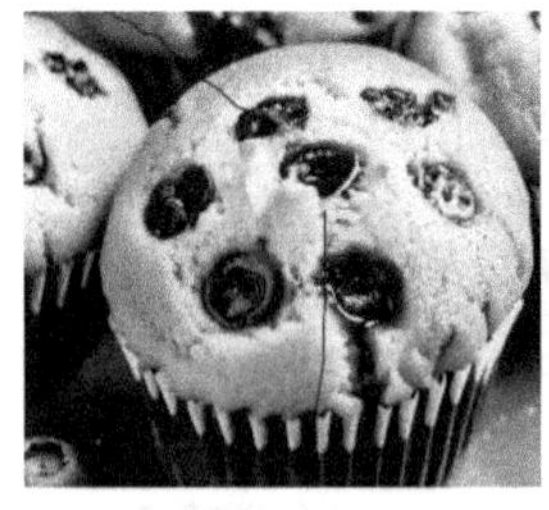

Almond Flour Blueberry Muffins

These moist and fluffy muffins are made with almond flour and bursting with juicy blueberries, perfect for a quick and satisfying dessert.

Preparation Time: 10 minutes
Cooking Time: 25 minutes
Total Time: 35 minutes
Servings: Makes 12 muffins

Ingredients

2 cups almond flour
1/4 cup coconut flour
1/4 cup coconut sugar
1 teaspoon baking powder
1/2 teaspoon baking soda
1/4 teaspoon salt
3 flax eggs (3 tablespoons ground flaxseed meal + 9 tablespoons water)
1/4 cup almond milk
1/4 cup melted coconut oil
1 teaspoon vanilla extract
1 cup fresh or frozen blueberries

Instructions

1. Preheat the oven to 350°F (175°C). Line a muffin tin with paper liners.
2. In a large mixing bowl, whisk together almond flour, coconut flour, coconut sugar, baking powder, baking soda, and salt.
3. In a separate bowl, prepare the flax eggs by mixing ground flaxseed meal with water.
4. Let sit for 5 minutes to thicken.
5. Stir almond milk, melted coconut oil, and vanilla extract into the flax eggs.
6. Add the wet ingredients to the dry ingredients and stir until just combined.
7. Gently fold in the blueberries.
8. Divide the batter evenly among the muffin cups.
9. Bake the muffins until golden brown and a toothpick inserted into the center comes out clean, for about 20-25 minutes.
10. Let cool in the tin for 5 minutes before transferring to a wire rack to cool completely.

Nutritional Info: Calories: 180, Protein: 5g, Carbohydrates: 15g, Fat: 12g, Fiber: 4g

Raw Vegan Chocolate Avocado Mousse

This creamy and decadent mousse is made with ripe avocados and rich cocoa powder for a guilt-free indulgence.

Preparation Time: 10 minutes
Cooking Time: 0 minutes
Total Time: 10 minutes
Servings: 2

Ingredients

2 ripe avocados
1/4 cup cocoa powder

1/4 cup maple syrup
1 teaspoon vanilla extract
Pinch of salt
Instructions
1. Scoop the flesh of the avocados into a blender or food processor.
2. Add cocoa powder, maple syrup, vanilla extract, and salt.
3. Blend until smooth and creamy, scraping down the sides as needed.
4. Divide the mousse into serving dishes.
5. Chill in the refrigerator for at least 30 minutes before serving.
Nutritional Info: Calories: 200, Protein: 3g, Carbohydrates: 20g, Fat: 15g, Fiber: 7g

Banana Nice Cream

This simple yet satisfying dessert is made by blending frozen bananas until smooth and creamy, resembling soft-serve ice cream.
Preparation Time: 5 minutes
Cooking Time: 0 minutes
Total Time: 5 minutes
Servings: 2
Ingredients
2 ripe bananas, sliced and frozen
Optional toppings: chopped nuts, shredded coconut, cacao nibs, fresh fruit
Instructions
1. Place frozen banana slices in a blender or food processor.
2. Blend until smooth and creamy, scraping down the sides as needed.
3. Serve immediately with your favorite toppings, if desired.
Nutritional Info: Calories: 150, Protein: 2g, Carbohydrates: 35g, Fat: 1g, Fiber: 4g

Coconut Chia Pudding

This creamy pudding is made with coconut milk and chia seeds, sweetened with a touch of maple syrup and flavored with vanilla.
Preparation Time: 5 minutes
Cooking Time: 0 minutes
Total Time: 5 minutes (+ chilling time)
Servings: 2
Ingredients
1 can (13.5 oz) full-fat coconut milk
1/4 cup chia seeds
2 tablespoons maple syrup
1 teaspoon vanilla extract
Instructions
1. In a mixing bowl, whisk together coconut milk, chia seeds, maple syrup, and vanilla extract.
2. Let the mixture sit for at least 5 minutes, then whisk again to avoid clumps.
3. Divide the mixture into serving glasses or jars.
4. Chill in the refrigerator for at least 2 hours, or overnight, until set.
Nutritional Info: Calories: 250, Protein: 4g, Carbohydrates: 20g, Fat: 18g, Fiber: 8g

Raw Vegan Key Lime Pie

This tangy and refreshing pie features a creamy avocado and cashew filling on a nutty date and almond crust, all naturally sweetened with maple syrup.

Preparation Time: 20 minutes

Cooking Time: 0 minutes

Total Time: 20 minutes (+ chilling time)

Servings: 8

Ingredients

For the crust:

1 cup raw almonds

1 cup pitted dates

Pinch of salt

For the filling:

2 ripe avocados

1/2 cup raw cashews (soaked for 4 hours or overnight)

1/2 cup freshly squeezed lime juice

1/4 cup maple syrup

1/4 cup coconut oil, melted

1 teaspoon lime zest

Pinch of salt

Instructions

1. In a food processor, pulse almonds, dates, and salt until the mixture sticks together when pressed.

2. Press the crust mixture evenly into the bottom of a pie pan.

3. In the same food processor (no need to clean it), blend together avocados, soaked cashews, lime juice, maple syrup, melted coconut oil, lime zest, and salt until smooth and creamy.

4. Pour the filling over the crust and smooth the top with a spatula.

5. Chill in the refrigerator for at least 4 hours, or until set.

6. Serve chilled, garnished with lime slices or zest, if desired.

Nutritional Info: Calories: 220, Protein: 4g, Carbohydrates: 25g, Fat: 15g, Fiber: 5g!

Quinoa Fruit Salad

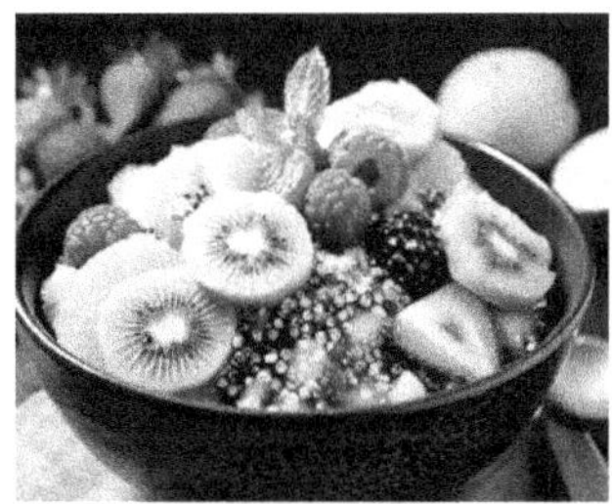

This refreshing fruit salad is enhanced with cooked quinoa for added texture and nutrition, making it a delightful dessert or snack.

Preparation Time: 15 minutes

Cooking Time: 15 minutes

Total Time: 30 minutes
Servings: Makes 4
Ingredients
1/2 cup quinoa, rinsed
1 cup water
2 cups mixed fruits (such as strawberries, blueberries, grapes, and kiwi), diced
2 tablespoons maple syrup
1 tablespoon lemon juice
1 teaspoon vanilla extract
Instructions
1. In a medium saucepan, bring water to a boil. Add quinoa, reduce heat, cover, and simmer for 15 minutes, or until quinoa is cooked and water is absorbed.
2. Remove from heat and let cool.
3. In a large mixing bowl, combine cooked quinoa and diced fruits.
4. In a small bowl, whisk together maple syrup, lemon juice, and vanilla extract.
5. Pour over the fruit and quinoa mixture, tossing gently to coat.
5. Chill in the refrigerator for at least 30 minutes before serving.
Nutritional Info: Calories: 150, Protein: 3g, Carbohydrates: 30g, Fat: 2g, Fiber: 4g

Almond Flour Carrot Cake Muffins

These fluffy muffins are loaded with shredded carrots and warm spices, making them a perfect plant-based dessert.
Preparation Time: 15 minutes
Cooking Time: 20 minutes
Total Time: 35 minutes
Servings: Makes 12 muffins
Ingredients
2 cups almond flour
1/4 cup coconut sugar
1 teaspoon baking powder
1/2 teaspoon baking soda
1/2 teaspoon ground cinnamon
1/4 teaspoon ground nutmeg
Pinch of salt
2 flax eggs (2 tablespoons ground flaxseed meal + 6 tablespoons water)
1/4 cup coconut oil, melted
1/4 cup almond milk
1 teaspoon vanilla extract
1 1/2 cups shredded carrots
1/4 cup chopped walnuts (optional)
Instructions
1. Preheat the oven to 350°F and line a muffin tin with paper liners.
2. in a large mixing bowl, whisk together almond flour, coconut sugar, baking powder, baking soda, cinnamon, nutmeg, and salt.
3. In a separate bowl, prepare the flax eggs by mixing ground flaxseed meal with water.

4. Let sit for 5 minutes to thicken.
5. Stir melted coconut oil, almond milk, and vanilla extract into the flax eggs.
6. Add the wet ingredients to the dry ingredients and stir until just combined.
7. Fold in shredded carrots and chopped walnuts, if using.
8. Divide the batter evenly among the muffin cups.
9. Bake for 18-20 minutes, or until a toothpick inserted into the center comes out clean.
10. Let cool in the tin for 5 minutes before transferring to a wire rack to cool completely.
Nutritional Info: Calories: 180, Protein: 5g, Carbohydrates: 15g, Fat: 12g, Fiber: 3g

Apple Walnut Crisp

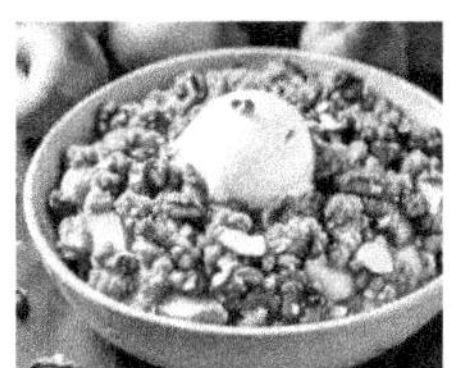

This comforting dessert features tender apples topped with a crunchy walnut crumble, making it a delightful treat for any occasion.
Preparation Time: 15 minutes
Cooking Time: 40 minutes
Total Time: 55 minutes
Servings: Makes 6
Ingredients
4 large apples, peeled, cored, and sliced
2 tablespoons maple syrup
1 tablespoon lemon juice
1 teaspoon ground cinnamon
1/2 cup almond flour
1/2 cup rolled oats (gluten-free)
1/4 cup chopped walnuts
2 tablespoons coconut oil, melted
2 tablespoons coconut sugar
Pinch of salt
Instructions
1. Preheat the oven to 350°F (175°C). Grease a baking dish with oil.
2. In a mixing bowl, toss sliced apples with maple syrup, lemon juice, and cinnamon.
3. Transfer to the prepared baking dish.
4. In a separate bowl, combine almond flour, rolled oats, chopped walnuts, melted coconut oil, coconut sugar, and salt. Mix until crumbly.
5. Sprinkle the walnut crumble evenly over the apples in the baking dish.
6. Bake for 35-40 minutes, or until the apples are tender and the topping is golden brown.
7. Let cool for a few minutes before serving.

Nutritional Info: Calories: 220, Protein: 4g, Carbohydrates: 30g, Fat: 10g, Fiber: 5g

Millet Chocolate Chip Cookies

These chewy chocolate chip cookies are made with nutritious millet flour for a wholesome and satisfying dessert.

Preparation Time: 15 minutes
Cooking Time: 10 minutes
Total Time: 25 minutes
Servings: Makes 12 cookies

Ingredients

1 cup millet flour
1/2 teaspoon baking soda
1/4 teaspoon salt
1/4 cup coconut oil, melted
1/4 cup maple syrup
1 flax egg (1 tablespoon ground flaxseed meal + 3 tablespoons water)
1 teaspoon vanilla extract
1/2 cup dairy-free chocolate chips

Instructions

1. Preheat the oven to 350°F and line a baking pan with parchment paper.
2. In a mixing bowl, whisk together millet flour, baking soda, and salt.
3. In a separate bowl, prepare the flax egg by mixing ground flaxseed meal with water.
4. Let it sit for 5 minutes to thicken.
5. Stir melted coconut oil, maple syrup, flax egg, and vanilla extract into the dry ingredients until well combined.
6. Fold in chocolate chips.
7. Drop spoonfuls of dough onto the prepared baking sheet and flatten slightly with the back of a spoon.
8. Bake for 8-10 minutes, or until the edges are golden brown.
9. Let cool on the baking sheet for 5 minutes before transferring to a wire rack to cool completely.

Nutritional Info: Calories: 150, Protein: 2g, Carbohydrates: 20g, Fat: 8g, Fiber: 2g

Carrot Cake Energy Balls

These bite-sized energy balls are reminiscent of carrot cake, featuring shredded carrots, walnuts, and warm spices for a nutritious dessert.

Preparation Time: 15 minutes
Cooking Time: 0 minutes
Total Time: 15 minutes
Servings: Makes 12 balls

Ingredients

1 cup rolled oats (gluten-free)
1/2 cup shredded carrots
1/4 cup chopped walnuts

1/4 cup raisins
2 tablespoons maple syrup
2 tablespoons almond butter
1 teaspoon ground cinnamon
1/2 teaspoon ground ginger
1/4 teaspoon ground nutmeg
Pinch of salt
Instructions
1. Place the rolled oat in a food processor bow and pulse until finely ground.
2. Add shredded carrots, chopped walnuts, raisins, maple syrup, almond butter, cinnamon, ginger, nutmeg, and salt.
3. Pulse until the mixture comes together and forms dough.
4. Roll the dough into small balls, about 1 tablespoon each.
5. Transfer to a baking sheet and lined with parchment paper.
6. Chill in the fridge for at least 30 minutes before serving.
Nutritional Info: Calories: 120, Protein: 3g, Carbohydrates: 15g, Fat: 6g, Fiber: 2g

Apple Walnut Oat Bars

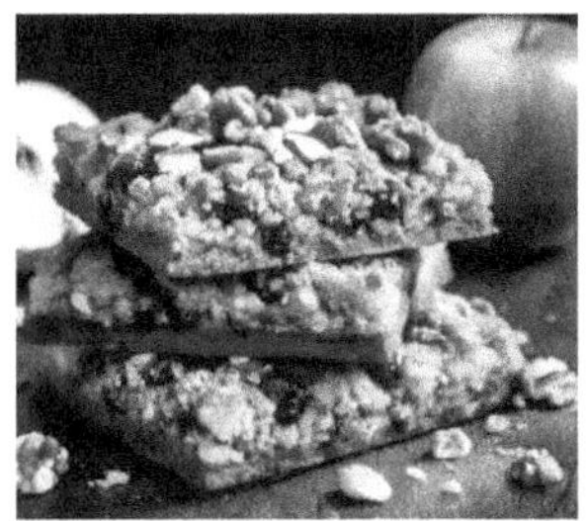

These hearty oat bars are packed with diced apples and crunchy walnuts, making them a perfect on-the-go dessert.
Preparation Time: 15 minutes
Cooking Time: 30 minutes
Total Time: 45 minutes
Servings: Makes 9 bars
Ingredients
1 1/2 cups rolled oats (gluten-free)
1 cup almond flour
1/4 cup coconut sugar
1 teaspoon ground cinnamon
1/2 teaspoon baking powder
Pinch of salt
1/4 cup coconut oil, melted
1/4 cup maple syrup
1 flax egg (1 tablespoon ground flaxseed meal + 3 tablespoons water)
1 teaspoon vanilla extract
1 large apple, peeled and diced
1/4 cup chopped walnuts
Instructions

1. Preheat the oven to 350°F (175°C). Line an 8x8-inch baking dish with parchment paper or Grease with oil.
2. In a large mixing bowl, combine rolled oats, almond flour, coconut sugar, cinnamon, baking powder, and salt.
3. In a separate bowl, prepare the flax egg by mixing ground flaxseed meal with water.
4. Let it sit for 5 minutes to thicken.
5. Stir melted coconut oil, maple syrup, flax egg, and vanilla extract into the dry ingredients until well combined.
6. Fold in diced apples and chopped walnuts.
7. Press the mixture evenly into the prepared baking dish.
8. Bake for 25-30 minutes, or until golden brown and set.
9. Let cool in the pan for 10 minutes before slicing into bars.
Nutritional Info: Calories: 200, Protein: 4g, Carbohydrates: 25g, Fat: 10g, Fiber: 4g

Millet Pudding with Mixed Berries

This creamy millet pudding is topped with a vibrant assortment of mixed berries for a luscious and satisfying dessert.
Preparation Time: 5 minutes
Cooking Time: 25 minutes
Total Time: 30 minutes (+ chilling time)
Servings: 4
Ingredients
1/2 cup millet
2 cups almond milk
1/4 cup maple syrup
1 teaspoon vanilla extract
Pinch of salt
1 cup mixed berries (such as blueberries, strawberries, and raspberries)
Instructions
1. Rinse millet under cold water and drain.
2. In a saucepan, combine millet, almond milk, maple syrup, vanilla extract, and salt.
3. Bring to a boil, then reduce heat and simmer, stirring occasionally, for 20-25 minutes, or until millet is tender and mixture has thickened.
4. Remove the saucepan from heat and let cool slightly.
5. Divide the millet pudding into serving bowls and top with mixed berries.
6. Chill in the refrigerator for at least 1 hour before serving.
Nutritional Info: Calories: 180, Protein: 3g, Carbohydrates: 30g, Fat: 5g, Fiber: 4g

Walnut Date Truffles

These decadent truffles are made with dates, walnuts, and a hint of vanilla for a naturally sweet and satisfying dessert.
Preparation Time: 15 minutes
Cooking Time: 0 minutes
Total Time: 15 minutes

Servings: Makes 12 truffles
Ingredients
1 cup pitted dates
1 cup walnuts
1 tablespoon almond butter
1 teaspoon vanilla extract
Pinch of salt
Shredded coconut or cocoa powder for coating (optional)
Instructions
1. In a food processor, pulse dates, walnuts, almond butter, vanilla extract, and salt until the mixture comes together and forms a dough.
2. Roll the dough into small balls, about 1 tablespoon each.
3. If desired, roll the truffles in shredded coconut or cocoa powder to coat.
4. Place in the fridge to chill for at least 30 minutes before serving
Nutritional Info: Calories: 120, Protein: 2g, Carbohydrates: 15g, Fat: 7g, Fiber: 2g

Apple Walnut Bread Pudding

This comforting bread pudding is studded with diced apples and chopped walnuts, making it a cozy and satisfying dessert for any occasion.
Preparation Time: 15 minutes
Cooking Time: 40 minutes
Total Time: 55 minutes
Servings: Makes 8
Ingredients
6 cups gluten-free bread cubes
2 large apples, peeled and diced
1/2 cup chopped walnuts
2 cups almond milk
1/4 cup maple syrup
2 flax eggs (2 tablespoons ground flaxseed meal + 6 tablespoons water)
1 teaspoon vanilla extract
1 teaspoon ground cinnamon
Pinch of salt
Instructions
1. Preheat the oven to 350°F (175°C). Grease a baking dish with coconut oil.
2. In a large mixing bowl, combine gluten-free bread cubes, diced apples, and chopped walnuts.
3. In a separate bowl, whisk together almond milk, maple syrup, flax eggs, vanilla extract, cinnamon, and salt.
4. Pour the wet mixture over the bread mixture, stirring until well combined.
5. Transfer the mixture to the prepared baking dish and evenly spreading it out evenly.
6. Bake for 35-40 minutes, or until golden brown.
7. Remove from the heat and let cool for a few minutes before serving.
Nutritional Info: Calories: 250, Protein: 5g, Carbohydrates: 35g, Fat: 10g, Fiber: 4g

Coconut Mango Nice Cream

This tropical-inspired nice cream is made with frozen bananas and mango for a refreshing and guilt-free dessert.

Preparation Time: 5 minutes
Cooking Time: 0 minutes
Total Time: 5 minutes
Servings: Makes 2

Ingredients

2 ripe bananas, sliced and frozen
1 cup frozen mango chunks
1/4 cup coconut milk

Instructions

1. In a blender or food processor, combine frozen bananas, frozen mango chunks, and coconut milk.
2. Blend until smooth and creamy, scraping down the sides as needed.
3. Serve immediately as soft-serve or transfer to a container and freeze for 1-2 hours for a firmer texture.

Nutritional Info: Calories: 150, Protein: 2g, Carbohydrates: 35g, Fat: 1g, Fiber: 5g

Quinoa Chocolate Chip Cookies

These chewy and satisfying cookies are made with quinoa flour and studded with chocolate chips for a delicious gluten-free treat.

Preparation Time: 15 minutes
Cooking Time: 12 minutes
Total Time: 27 minutes
Servings: Makes 16 cookies

Ingredients

1 cup quinoa flour
1/2 teaspoon baking soda
1/4 teaspoon salt
1/4 cup coconut oil, melted
1/4 cup maple syrup
1 flax egg (1 tablespoon ground flaxseed meal + 3 tablespoons water)
1 teaspoon vanilla extract
1/2 cup dairy-free chocolate chips

Instructions

1. Preheat the oven to 350°F and line a baking sheet with parchment paper or grease with oil.
2. In a mixing large bowl, whisk together baking soda, quinoa flour, and salt.
3. In a separate bowl, prepare the flax egg by mixing ground flaxseed meal with water.
4. Let it sit for 5 minutes to thicken.
5. Stir melted coconut oil, maple syrup, flax egg, and vanilla extract into the dry ingredients until well combined.
6. Fold in chocolate chips.

7. Drop spoonfuls of dough onto the prepared baking sheet and flatten slightly with the back of a spoon.
8. Place in the heated oven bake for 10-12 minutes, or until the edges are golden brown.
9. Remove from the oven and let cool on a baking sheet for 5 minutes before transferring to a wire rack to completely cool.
Nutritional Info: Calories: 150, Protein: 2g, Carbohydrates: 20g, Fat: 8g, Fiber: 2g

Chia Seed Pudding with Mixed Berries

This creamy chia seed pudding is topped with a vibrant assortment of mixed berries for a refreshing and nutritious dessert.
Preparation Time: 5 minutes
Cooking Time: 0 minutes
Total Time: 5 minutes (+ chilling time)
Servings: Makes 2
Ingredients
1/4 cup chia seeds
1 cup almond milk
1 tablespoon maple syrup (optional)
1/2 cup mixed berries (such as strawberries, raspberries and blueberries)
Instructions
1. In a bowl, whisk together chia seeds, almond milk, and maple syrup (if using).
2. Let the mixture sit for 5 minutes, then whisk again to prevent clumping.
3. Cover and refrigerate for at least 2 hours or overnight, until the pudding thickens.
4. Before serving, divide the chia seed pudding into serving glasses and top with mixed berries.
Nutritional Info: Calories: 120, Protein: 4g, Carbohydrates: 15g, Fat: 5g, Fiber: 8g

Frozen Banana Bites

These frozen banana bites are coated in chocolate and topped with various toppings for a fun and customizable dessert.
Preparation Time: 10 minutes
Cooking Time: 0 minutes
Total Time: 10 minutes (+ freezing time)
Servings: 12 bites
Ingredients
2 large ripe bananas, peeled and sliced into rounds
1/2 cup dairy-free chocolate chips
2 tablespoons coconut oil
Toppings of your choice (such as shredded coconut, chopped nuts, or dried fruit)
Instructions
1. Place banana slices on a parchment-lined baking sheet and freeze for 1-2 hours, until firm.
2. In a microwave-safe bowl, combine the oil and chocolate chips.
3. Microwave in 30-second intervals, stirring until smooth.

4. Using a fork, dip each frozen banana slice into the melted chocolate, coating it completely.

5. Place the chocolate-coated banana slice back onto the parchment-lined baking sheet and sprinkle with toppings.

6. Return the baking sheet to the freezer and freeze for an additional 30 minutes, until the chocolate is set.

Nutritional Info: Calories: 90, Protein: 1g, Carbohydrates: 10g, Fat: 6g, Fiber: 2g

Peanut Butter Protein Balls

These protein-packed balls are made with peanut butter, oats, and chia seeds for a satisfying and energizing dessert.

Preparation Time: 10 minutes

Cooking Time: 0 minutes

Total Time: 10 minutes

Servings: Makes 12 balls

Ingredients

1 cup rolled oats (gluten-free)

1/2 cup creamy peanut butter

1/4 cup maple syrup

2 tablespoons chia seeds

1 teaspoon vanilla extract

Pinch of salt

Instructions

1. In a mixing bowl, combine rolled oats, peanut butter, maple syrup, chia seeds, vanilla extract, and salt.

2. Stir until well combined and the mixture holds together.

3. Roll the mixture into small balls and place them on a parchment-lined baking sheet.

4. Place in the fridge to chill for at least 30 minutes before serving.

Nutritional Info: Calories: 130, Protein: 4g, Carbohydrates: 12g, Fat: 8g, Fiber: 2g

Berry Coconut Parfait

This layered parfait combines creamy coconut yogurt with fresh berries and crunchy granola for a delightful and satisfying dessert.

Preparation Time: 5 minutes

Cooking Time: 0 minutes

Total Time: 5 minutes

Servings: 2

Ingredients

1 cup coconut yogurt

1/2 cup mixed berries (such as strawberries, raspberries and blueberries,)

1/4 cup gluten-free granola

Instructions

1. In two serving glasses, layer coconut yogurt, mixed berries, and granola.

2. Repeat the layers until the glasses are filled.

3. Refrigerate until ready to serve or serve immediately.

Chocolate Covered Strawberries

These classic chocolate-covered strawberries are a simple yet elegant dessert that's perfect for any occasion.

Preparation Time: 10 minutes
Cooking Time: 0 minutes
Total Time: 10 minutes (+ chilling time)
Servings: Makes 12 strawberries

Ingredients

12 large strawberries, washed and dried
1/2 cup dairy-free chocolate chips
1 teaspoon coconut oil

Instructions

1. Line a baking sheet with parchment paper.
2. In a microwave-safe bowl, combine oil and chocolate chips.
3. Microwave in 30-second intervals, stirring until smooth.
4. Dip each strawberry into the melted chocolate, coating it halfway.
5. Place the chocolate-covered strawberries onto the prepared baking sheet.
6. Chill in the refrigerator for at least 30 minutes, until the chocolate is set.

Nutritional Info: Calories: 60, Protein: 1g, Carbohydrates: 10g, Fat: 3g, Fiber: 2g

Apple Cinnamon Baked Oatmeal Cups

These baked oatmeal cups are flavored with apple and cinnamon for a comforting and nutritious dessert.

Preparation Time: 10 minutes
Cooking Time: 25 minutes
Total Time: 35 minutes
Servings: Makes 12 cups

Ingredients

2 cups rolled oats (gluten-free)
1 teaspoon baking powder
1/2 teaspoon ground cinnamon
1/4 teaspoon salt
1 1/2 cups almond milk
1/4 cup maple syrup
1 teaspoon vanilla extract
1 apple, peeled and diced

Instructions

1. Preheat the oven to 350°F (175°C) and grease a muffin tin or parchment paper.
2. In a mixing bowl, combine rolled oats, baking powder, cinnamon, and salt.
3. in a separate bowl, whisk together almond milk, maple syrup, and vanilla extract.
4. Pour the wet ingredients into the bowl of dry ingredients and stir to combine.
5. Fold in diced apple.
6. Divide the mixture equally among the muffin cups.
7. Bake for 25 minutes, or until golden brown and set.

8. Let cool before serving.

Nutritional Info: Calories: 120, Protein: 3g, Carbohydrates: 20g, Fat: 3g, Fiber: 2g

STEW

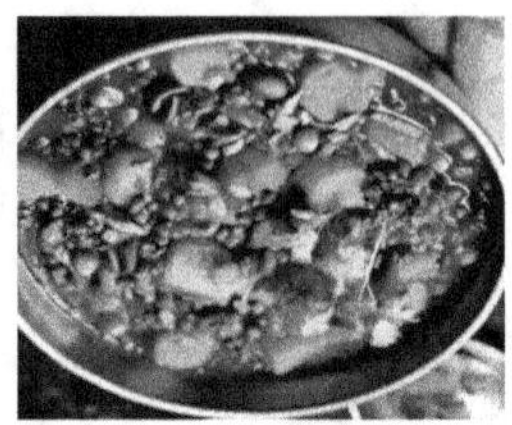

Vegetable Lentil Stew

A hearty and nutritious stew packed with vegetables and protein-rich lentils.
Preparation Time: 15 minutes
Cooking Time: 30 minutes
Total Time: 45 minutes
Servings: 4
Ingredients
1 cup green or brown lentils, rinsed
4 cups vegetable broth
2 carrots, diced
2 celery stalks, diced
1 onion, diced
2 garlic cloves, minced
1 teaspoon dried thyme
1 teaspoon paprika
Salt and pepper to taste
Fresh parsley for garnish (optional)
Instructions
1. In a large pot, combine lentils, vegetable broth, carrots, celery, onion, garlic, thyme, and paprika.
2. Bring to a boil, then reduce heat and simmer for 25-30 minutes until lentils and vegetables are tender.
3. Season the stew with salt and pepper to taste.
4. Serve hot, garnished with fresh parsley if desired.
Nutritional Info: Calories: 250, Protein: 15g, Carbohydrates: 45g, Fat: 2g, Fiber: 15g

Chickpea and Spinach Stew

A comforting stew with chickpeas, spinach, and aromatic spices.
Preparation Time: 15 minutes
Cooking Time: 25 minutes
Total Time: 40 minutes
Servings: 4
Ingredients
2 cans (15 oz. each) chickpeas, drained and rinsed
1 onion, diced
3 garlic cloves, minced
1 teaspoon ground cumin
1 teaspoon ground coriander
1/2 teaspoon smoked paprika
1/4 teaspoon cayenne pepper (optional)
4 cups vegetable broth
4 cups fresh spinach leaves
Salt and pepper to taste
Instructions
1. In a large pot, sauté onion and garlic over medium heat until softened.

2. Add ground cumin, ground coriander, smoked paprika, and cayenne pepper. Stir well to combine.

3. Add chickpeas and vegetable broth. Bring to a simmer and cook for 15 minutes.

4. Add fresh spinach leaves and cook for an additional 5 minutes until wilted.

5. Season the stew with salt and pepper to taste.

6. Serve hot.

Nutritional Info: Calories: 280, Protein: 14g, Carbohydrates: 46g, Fat: 4g, Fiber: 13g

Coconut Curry Lentil Stew

A creamy and flavorful stew with lentils, vegetables, and aromatic curry spices.

Preparation Time: 15 minutes

Cooking Time: 35 minutes

Total Time: 50 minutes

Serving: 4

Ingredients

1 cup red lentils, rinsed

1 onion, diced

2 garlic cloves, minced

1 tablespoon curry powder

1 teaspoon ground turmeric

1 can (14 oz) coconut milk

3 cups vegetable broth

2 cups chopped tomatoes

2 cups chopped spinach

Salt and pepper to taste

Fresh cilantro for garnish (optional)

Instructions

1. In a large pot, sauté onion and garlic until softened.

2. Add curry powder and ground turmeric. Stir for 1 minute.

3. Add red lentils, coconut milk, vegetable broth, and chopped tomatoes.

4. Bring to a boil, then reduce heat and simmer for 25-30 minutes until lentils are tender.

5. Stir in chopped spinach and cook for an additional 5 minutes until wilted.

6. Season with salt and pepper to taste.

7. Serve hot, garnished with fresh cilantro if desired.

Nutritional Info: Calories: 320, Protein: 15g, Carbohydrates: 40g, Fat: 12g, Fiber: 14g

Quinoa and Vegetable Stew

A protein-packed stew with quinoa, mixed vegetables, and savory herbs.

Preparation Time: 15 minutes

Cooking Time: 25 minutes

Total Time: 40 minutes

Servings: 4

Ingredients

1 cup quinoa, rinsed

4 cups vegetable broth

1 onion, diced
2 carrots, diced
2 celery stalks, diced
1 bell pepper, diced
2 garlic cloves, minced
1 teaspoon dried thyme
1 teaspoon dried rosemary
Salt and pepper to taste
Fresh parsley for garnish (optional)

Instructions

1. In a large pot, combine quinoa, vegetable broth, onion, carrots, celery, bell pepper, garlic, dried thyme, and dried rosemary.
2. Bring to a boil, then reduce heat and simmer for 20-25 minutes until quinoa and vegetables are tender.
3. Season with salt and pepper to taste.
4. Serve hot, garnished with fresh parsley if desired.

Nutritional Info: Calories: 290, Protein: 11g, Carbohydrates: 50g, Fat: 4g, Fiber: 8g

Sweet Potato and Black Bean Stew

A comforting stew with sweet potatoes, black beans, and warming spices.

Preparation Time: 15 minutes
Cooking Time: 30 minutes
Total Time: 45 minutes
Servings: 4

Ingredients:

2 large sweet potatoes, peeled and diced
1 onion, diced
2 garlic cloves, minced
1 teaspoon ground cumin
1 teaspoon smoked paprika
1/4 teaspoon chili powder (optional)
2 cans black beans (15 oz. each) drained and rinsed
1 can (14 oz) diced tomatoes
4 cups vegetable broth
Salt and pepper to taste
Fresh cilantro for garnish (optional)

Instruction

1. 1In a large pot, sauté onion and garlic until softened.
2. Add diced sweet potatoes, ground cumin, smoked paprika, and chili powder (if using).
3. Stir well to coat.
4. Add black beans, diced tomatoes, and vegetable broth.
5. Bring to a boil, then reduce heat and simmer for 20-25 minutes until sweet potatoes are tender.
6. Season with salt and pepper to taste.
7. Serve hot, garnished with fresh cilantro if desired.

Nutritional Info: Calories: 280, Protein: 12g, Carbohydrates: 50g, Fat: 2g, Fiber: 15g

Butternut Squash and Kale Stew

A comforting stew with creamy butternut squash, hearty kale, and aromatic spices.
Preparation Time: 20 minutes
Cooking Time: 25 minutes
Total Time: 45 minutes
Servings: 4
Ingredients
1 small butternut squash, peeled, seeded, and diced
1 onion, diced
2 garlic cloves, minced
1 teaspoon ground cumin
1/2 teaspoon ground cinnamon
4 cups vegetable broth
4 cups chopped kale leaves
Salt and pepper to taste
Toasted pumpkin seeds for garnish (optional)
Instructions
1. In a large pot, sauté onion and garlic until softened.
2. Add diced butternut squash, ground cumin, and ground cinnamon. Stir well to coat.
3. Add vegetable broth and let it boil.
4. Reduce heat and simmer for 15-20 minutes until squash is tender.
5. Add chopped kale leaves and cook for an additional 5 minutes until wilted.
6. Season with salt and pepper to taste.
7. Serve hot, garnished with toasted pumpkin seeds if desired.
Nutritional Info: Calories: 220, Protein: 8g, Carbohydrates: 45g, Fat: 2g, Fiber: 10g

Spicy Three-Bean Stew

A spicy and satisfying stew with three varieties of beans and bold flavors.
Preparation Time: 15 minutes
Cooking Time: 35 minutes
Total Time: 50 minutes
Servings: 4
Ingredients
1 can black beans (15 oz.) drained and rinsed
1 can kidney beans (15 oz.) drained and rinsed
1 can chickpeas (15 oz.) drained and rinsed
1 onion, diced
2 garlic cloves, minced
1 bell pepper, diced
1 jalapeño pepper, seeded and minced
1 tablespoon chili powder
1 teaspoon ground cumin
1/2 teaspoon smoked paprika

1 can (14 oz) diced tomatoes
4 cups vegetable broth
Salt and pepper to taste
Fresh cilantro for garnish (optional)
Instructions
1. In a large pot, sauté onion, garlic, bell pepper, and jalapeño pepper until softened.
2. Add chili powder, ground cumin, and smoked paprika. Stir well to coat.
3. Add black beans, kidney beans, chickpeas, diced tomatoes, and vegetable broth.
4. Bring to a boil, then reduce heat to low and let it simmer for about 25-30 minutes.
5. Season with salt and pepper to taste.
6. Garnished with fresh cilantro if desired and serve immediately
Nutritional Info: Calories: 320, Protein: 16g, Carbohydrates: 55g, Fat: 2g, Fiber: 18g

Mushroom and Barley Stew

A hearty and earthy stew with tender mushrooms, barley, and aromatic herbs.
Preparation Time: 20 minutes
Cooking Time: 40 minutes
Total Time: 1 hour
Servings: 4
Ingredients
1 cup pearl barley, rinsed
4 cups vegetable broth
1 onion, diced
2 garlic cloves, minced
8 oz mushrooms, sliced
2 carrots, diced
2 celery stalks, diced
1 teaspoon dried thyme
1 teaspoon dried rosemary
Salt and pepper to taste
Fresh parsley for garnish (optional)
Instructions
1. In a large pot, combine pearl barley, vegetable broth, onion, garlic, mushrooms, carrots, celery, dried thyme, and dried rosemary.
2. Bring to a boil, then reduce heat and simmer for 30-35 minutes until barley and vegetables are tender.
3. Season with salt and pepper to taste.
4. Serve hot, garnished with fresh parsley if desired.
Nutritional Info: Calories: 290, Protein: 10g, Carbohydrates: 55g, Fat: 2g, Fiber: 12g

Moroccan Chickpea Tagine

A fragrant and exotic stew with chickpeas, vegetables, and Moroccan spices.
Preparation Time: 20 minutes
Cooking Time: 40 minutes

Total Time: 1 hour
Servings: 4
Ingredients
2 cans (15 oz each) chickpeas, drained and rinsed
1 onion, diced
2 garlic cloves, minced
1 teaspoon ground cumin
1 teaspoon ground coriander
1/2 teaspoon ground cinnamon
1/4 teaspoon ground ginger
1/4 teaspoon cayenne pepper
1 can (14 oz) diced tomatoes
2 cups vegetable broth
1 cup chopped dried apricots
Salt and pepper to taste
Fresh cilantro for garnish (optional)
Instructions
1. In a large pot, sauté onion and garlic until softened.
2. Add ground cumin, ground coriander, ground cinnamon, ground ginger, and cayenne pepper. Stir well to coat.
3. Add chickpeas, diced tomatoes, vegetable broth, and chopped dried apricots.
4. Bring to a boil, then reduce heat and simmer for 30-35 minutes.
5. Season with salt and pepper to taste.
6. Garnished with fresh cilantro if you want and serve immediately
Nutritional Info: Calories: 320, Protein: 14g, Carbohydrates: 55g, Fat: 2g, Fiber: 14g
Red Lentil and Vegetable Stew
A nourishing stew with red lentils, colorful vegetables, and warming spices.

Preparation Time: 15 minutes

Cooking Time: 25 minutes
Total Time: 40 minutes
Servings: 4
Ingredients
1 cup red lentils, rinsed
4 cups vegetable broth
1 onion, diced
2 carrots, diced
2 celery stalks, diced
1 bell pepper, diced
2 garlic cloves, minced
1 teaspoon ground cumin
1 teaspoon smoked paprika
Salt and pepper to taste
Fresh parsley for garnish (optional)
Instructions

1. In a large pot, combine red lentils, vegetable broth, onion, carrots, celery, bell pepper, garlic, ground cumin, and smoked paprika.
2. Bring to a boil, then reduce heat and simmer for 20-25 minutes until lentils and vegetables are tender.
3. Season with salt and pepper to taste.
4. Serve hot, garnished with fresh parsley if desired.
Nutritional Info: Calories: 270, Protein: 15g, Carbohydrates: 45g, Fat: 2g, Fiber: 12g

Potato and Leek Stew

A comforting and creamy stew with tender potatoes, leeks, and savory herbs.
Preparation Time: 20 minutes
Cooking Time: 35 minutes
Total Time: 55 minutes
Servings: 4
Ingredients
4 large potatoes, peeled and diced
2 leeks, white and light green parts only, sliced
1 onion, diced
2 garlic cloves, minced
4 cups vegetable broth
1 teaspoon dried thyme
1 teaspoon dried rosemary
1/2 cup coconut cream or full-fat coconut milk
Salt and pepper to taste
Fresh chives for garnish (optional)
Instructions
1. In a large pot, sauté leeks, onion, and garlic until softened.
2. Add diced potatoes, vegetable broth, dried thyme, and dried rosemary.
3. Bring to a boil, then reduce heat and simmer for 25-30 minutes until potatoes are tender.
4. Stir in coconut cream or coconut milk and cook for an additional 5 minutes.
5. Season with salt and pepper to taste.
6. Serve hot, garnished with fresh chives if desired.
Nutritional Info: Calories: 320, Protein: 7g, Carbohydrates: 50g, Fat: 10g, Fiber: 8g

Tomato and White Bean Stew

A simple and comforting stew with tomatoes, white beans, and Italian herbs.
Preparation Time: 15 minutes
Cooking Time: 25 minutes
Total Time: 40 minutes
Servings: 4
Ingredients
2 cans (15 oz each) white beans, drained and rinsed
1 onion, diced
2 garlic cloves, minced
1 can (14 oz) diced tomatoes

2 cups vegetable broth
1 teaspoon dried oregano
1 teaspoon dried basil
Salt and pepper to taste
Fresh basil for garnish (optional)

Instructions

1. In a large pot, sauté onion and garlic until softened.
2. Add white beans, diced tomatoes, vegetable broth, dried oregano, and dried basil.
3. Bring to a boil, then reduce heat and simmer for 20-25 minutes.
4. Season the stew with salt and pepper to taste.
5. Serve hot, garnished with fresh basil if desired.

Nutritional Info: Calories: 250, Protein: 10g, Carbohydrates: 40g, Fat: 2g, Fiber: 12g

Spicy Lentil and Kale Stew

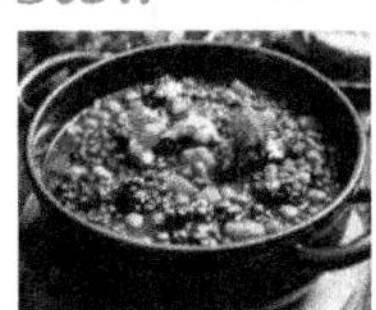

A spicy and nutritious stew with lentils, kale, and bold spices.
Preparation Time: 20 minutes
Cooking Time: 30 minutes
Total Time: 50 minutes
Servings: 4

Ingredients

1 cup green or brown lentils, rinsed
4 cups vegetable broth
1 onion, diced
2 garlic cloves, minced
1 bell pepper, diced
1 jalapeño pepper, seeded and minced
2 cups chopped kale leaves
1 teaspoon ground cumin
1 teaspoon smoked paprika
Salt and pepper to taste
Fresh cilantro for garnish (optional)

Instructions

1. In a large pot, sauté onion, garlic, bell pepper, and jalapeño pepper until softened.
2. Add lentils, vegetable broth, chopped kale leaves, ground cumin, and smoked paprika.
3. Bring to a boil, then reduce heat and simmer for 25-30 minutes until lentils are tender.
4. Season the stew with salt and pepper to taste.
5. Garnished with fresh cilantro if desired, serve immediately,

Nutritional Info: Calories: 280, Protein: 16g, Carbohydrates: 45g, Fat: 2g, Fiber: 15g

Indian Spiced Cauliflower Stew

A flavorful and aromatic stew with cauliflower, chickpeas, and Indian spices.
Preparation Time: 20 minutes
Cooking Time: 35 minutes
Total Time: 55 minutes
Servings: 4
Ingredients
1 head cauliflower, cut into florets
1 onion, diced
2 garlic cloves, minced
1 tablespoon curry powder
1 teaspoon ground cumin
1 teaspoon ground coriander
1/2 teaspoon ground turmeric
1/4 teaspoon cayenne pepper (optional)
1 can (15 oz) chickpeas, drained and rinsed
1 can (14 oz) diced tomatoes
4 cups vegetable broth
Salt and pepper to taste
Fresh cilantro for garnish (optional)
Instructions
1. In a large pot, sauté onion and garlic until softened.
2. Add curry powder, ground cumin, ground coriander, ground turmeric, and cayenne pepper (if using).
3. Stir well to coat.
4. Add cauliflower florets, chickpeas, diced tomatoes, and vegetable broth.
5. Bring to a boil, then reduce heat and simmer for 30-35 minutes until cauliflower is tender.
6. Season with salt and pepper to taste.
7. Serve hot, garnished with fresh cilantro if desired.
Nutritional Info: Calories: 290, Protein: 12g, Carbohydrates: 45g, Fat: 2g, Fiber: 14g

Rainbow Chard and White Bean Stew

A vibrant and nutritious stew with rainbow chard, white beans, and aromatic herbs.
Preparation Time: 20 minutes
Cooking Time: 25 minutes
Total Time: 45 minutes
Servings: 4
Ingredients
1 bunch rainbow chard, stems removed, leaves chopped
1 onion, diced
2 garlic cloves, minced
2 cans (15 oz each) white beans, drained and rinsed
1 can (14 oz) diced tomatoes
4 cups vegetable broth
1 teaspoon dried thyme

1 teaspoon dried basil

Salt and pepper to taste

Fresh parsley for garnish (optional)

Instructions

1. In a large pot, sauté onion and garlic until softened.

2. Add chopped rainbow chard leaves and cook until wilted.

3. Add white beans, diced tomatoes, vegetable broth, dried thyme, and dried basil.

4. Bring to a boil, then reduce heat and simmer for 20-25 minutes.

5. Season with salt and pepper to taste.

6. Serve hot, garnished with fresh parsley if desired.

Nutritional Info: Calories: 270, Protein: 15g, Carbohydrates: 45g, Fat: 2g, Fiber: 12g

Cauliflower Chickpea Stew

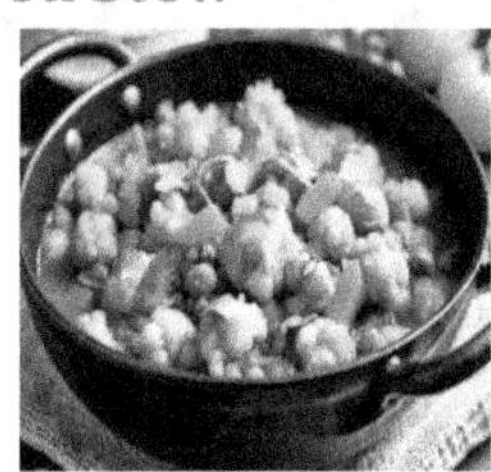

A hearty and satisfying stew with cauliflower, chickpeas, and warming spices.

Preparation Time: 15 minutes

Cooking Time: 30 minutes

Total Time: 45 minutes

Servings: 4

Ingredients

1 cauliflower, cut into florets

1 onion, diced

2 cloves garlic, minced

1 can (14 oz) diced tomatoes

1 can (14 oz) chickpeas, drained and rinsed

2 cups vegetable broth

1 teaspoon ground cumin

1 teaspoon ground turmeric

1/2 teaspoon ground coriander

Salt and pepper to taste

Fresh parsley for garnish (optional)

Instructions

1. In a large pot, combine cauliflower florets, diced onion, minced garlic, diced tomatoes, chickpeas, vegetable broth, ground cumin, ground turmeric, and ground coriander.

2. Bring to a boil, then reduce heat to low and simmer for 25-30 minutes, or until cauliflower is tender.

3. Season with salt and pepper to taste.

4. Serve hot, garnished with fresh parsley if desired.

Nutritional Info: Calories: 250, Protein: 11g, Carbohydrates: 45g, Fat: 3g, Fiber: 14g

Red Lentil Coconut Stew

A creamy and aromatic stew with red lentils, coconut milk, and warming spices.
Preparation Time: 15 minutes
Cooking Time: 25 minutes
Total Time: 40 minutes
Servings: 4
Ingredients
1 cup red lentils, rinsed
1 can (14 oz) coconut milk
1 onion, diced
2 cloves garlic, minced
1 bell pepper, diced
1 tablespoon curry powder
1 teaspoon ground turmeric
1/2 teaspoon ground cumin
Salt and pepper to taste
Fresh cilantro for garnish (optional)
Instructions
1. In a large pot, combine red lentils, coconut milk, diced onion, minced garlic, diced bell pepper, curry powder, ground turmeric, and ground cumin.
2 Bring to a boil, then reduce heat to low and simmer for 20-25 minutes, stirring occasionally, until lentils are tender and the stew has thickened.
3. Season with salt and pepper to taste.
4. Serve hot, garnished with fresh cilantro if desired.
Nutritional Info: Calories: 250, Protein: 12g, Carbohydrates: 34g, Fat: 8g, Fiber: 13g

Spicy Mushroom and Tofu Hot Pot

Fragrant stew with mushrooms, tofu, and Chinese herbs and spices.
Preparation Time: 20 minutes
Cooking Time: 30 minutes
Total Time: 50 minutes
Servings: 4
Ingredients
1 block (14 oz) firm tofu, cubed
2 cups mixed mushrooms (such as shiitake, cremini, oyster), sliced
1 onion, sliced
3 cloves garlic, minced
1 tablespoon soy sauce or tamari
1 tablespoon rice vinegar
1 teaspoon sesame oil
4 cups vegetable broth
2 tablespoons miso paste
1 tablespoon grated ginger
2 green onions, sliced

Instructions

1. In a large pot, sauté tofu cubes until golden brown. Set aside.
2. In the same pot, sauté onion and garlic until softened.
3. Add mixed mushrooms, soy sauce, rice vinegar, sesame oil, vegetable broth, miso paste, and grated ginger.
4. Simmer for 20-25 minutes until mushrooms are tender.
5. Stir in cooked tofu and sliced green onions.
6. Serve hot, garnished with additional sliced green onions if desired.
Nutritional Info: Calories: 250, Protein: 18g, Carbohydrates: 20g, Fat: 10g, Fiber: 6g

Chinese-Inspired Vegetable and Tofu Miso Stew

Flavorful stew with tofu, assorted vegetables, and miso paste.
Preparation Time: 20 minutes
Cooking Time: 30 minutes
Total Time: 50 minutes
Servings: 4
Ingredients
1 block (14 oz) firm tofu, cubed
2 cups mixed vegetables (such as carrots, broccoli, and snap peas)
1 onion, sliced
3 cloves garlic, minced
2 tablespoons soy sauce or tamari
4 cups vegetable broth
2 tablespoons miso paste
1 tablespoon grated ginger
2 green onions, sliced
Instructions

1. In a large pot, sauté tofu cubes until golden brown. Set aside.
2. In the same pot, sauté onion and garlic until softened.
3. Add mixed vegetables, soy sauce, vegetable broth, miso paste, and grated ginger.
4. Simmer for 20-25 minutes until vegetables are tender.
5. Stir in cooked tofu and sliced green onions.
6. Serve hot, garnished with additional sliced green onions if desired.
Nutritional Info: Calories: 250, Protein: 16g, Carbohydrates: 20g, Fat: 12g, Fiber: 6g

Chinese Spiced Eggplant and Tofu Stew

Flavorful stew with eggplant, tofu, and Chinese seasonings.
Preparation Time: 20 minutes
Cooking Time: 30 minutes
Total Time: 50 minutes
Servings: 4
Ingredients
1 block (14 oz) firm tofu, cubed
2 Japanese eggplants, sliced
1 onion, sliced
3 cloves garlic, minced

2 tablespoons soy sauce or tamari

1 tablespoon rice vinegar

1 teaspoon sesame oil

1 teaspoon grated ginger

4 cups vegetable broth

1 tablespoon cornstarch (or arrowroot powder) mixed with 2 tablespoons water (for thickening)

Instructions

1. In a large pot, sauté tofu cubes until golden brown. Set aside.

2. In the same pot, sauté onion and garlic until softened.

3. Add eggplant slices, soy sauce, rice vinegar, sesame oil, grated ginger, and vegetable broth.

4. Simmer for 20-25 minutes until eggplant is tender.

5. Stir in the cornstarch mixture and cooked tofu, and simmer for another 5 minutes until thickened.

6. Serve hot over cooked rice or noodles.

Nutritional Info: Calories: 280, Protein: 16g, Carbohydrates: 25g, Fat: 10g, Fiber: 8g

Mexican Stew with corn and potato

Comforting stew with corn, potatoes, and Mexican spices.

Preparation Time: 15 minutes

Cooking Time: 30 minutes

Total Time: 45 minutes

Servings: 6

Ingredients

4 potatoes, peeled and diced

2 cups frozen corn kernels

1 onion, chopped

3 cloves garlic, minced

1 can (14 oz) diced tomatoes

4 cups vegetable broth

1 tablespoon chili powder

1 teaspoon cumin

1/2 teaspoon smoked paprika

Salt and pepper to taste

Instructions

1. In a large pot, sauté onion and garlic until softened.

2. Add diced potatoes, frozen corn kernels, diced tomatoes, vegetable broth, chili powder, cumin, smoked paprika, salt, and pepper.

3. Simmer for 25-30 minutes until potatoes are tender.

4. Garnished with chopped cilantro if you want and serve hot.

Nutritional Info: Calories: 240, Protein: 6g, Carbohydrates: 50g, Fat: 1g, Fiber: 8g

Mexican-Inspired Pumpkin and Black Bean Stew

Comforting stew with pumpkin, black beans, and Mexican spices.

Preparation Time: 20 minutes

Cooking Time: 35 minutes
Total Time: 55 minutes
Servings: 6
Ingredients
2 cups pumpkin, peeled and diced
1 onion, chopped
3 cloves garlic, minced
1 bell pepper, diced
1 can (15 oz) black beans, drained and rinsed
1 can (14 oz) diced tomatoes
4 cups vegetable broth
1 tablespoon chili powder
1 teaspoon cumin
1/2 teaspoon smoked paprika
Salt and pepper to taste
Instructions
1. In a large pot, sauté onion and garlic until softened.
2. Add diced pumpkin, bell pepper, black beans, diced tomatoes, vegetable broth, chili powder, cumin, smoked paprika, salt, and pepper.
3. Simmer for 30-35 minutes until pumpkin is tender.
4. Garnished with chopped cilantro if you want and serve hot.
Nutritional Info: Calories: 260, Protein: 10g, Carbohydrates: 50g, Fat: 1g, Fiber: 12g

DRESSINGS

Tahini Lemon Herb

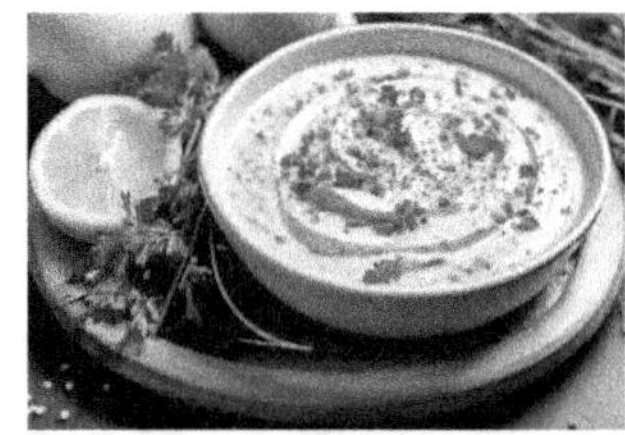

A creamy and tangy dressing with the richness of tahini and the freshness of herbs and lemon.
Preparation Time: 5 minutes
Total Time: 5 minutes
Serving: 3/4 cup
Ingredients
1/4 cup tahini
Juice of 1 lemon
2 tablespoons chopped fresh parsley
2 tablespoons chopped fresh cilantro
1 garlic clove, minced
Water, as needed

Instructions
1. In a small bowl, whisk together tahini, lemon juice, chopped fresh parsley, chopped fresh cilantro, and minced garlic until smooth.
2. Thin the dressing with water to reach desired consistency.
3. Serve immediately over salads or store in an airtight container in the refrigerator for up to one week.
Nutritional Info: Calories: 90, Protein: 3g, Carbohydrates: 5g, Fat: 7g, Fiber: 2g

Cashew Caesar Dressing

A creamy and indulgent dressing with the richness of cashews and classic Caesar flavors.
Preparation Time: 10 minutes
Total Time: 10 minutes
Serving: 1 cup
Ingredients
1/2 cup raw cashews, soaked for at least 2 hours
2 tablespoons nutritional yeast
Juice of 1 lemon
1 tablespoon Dijon mustard
1 garlic clove, minced
Water, as needed
Instructions
1. In a blender, combine soaked cashews, nutritional yeast, lemon juice, Dijon mustard, and minced garlic.
2. Blend until smooth, adding water as needed to reach desired consistency.
3. Serve immediately over salads or store in an airtight container in the refrigerator for up to one week.
Nutritional Info: Calories: 120, Protein: 5g, Carbohydrates: 7g, Fat: 9g, Fiber: 2g

Walnut Pesto Dressing

A flavorful and nutty dressing with the richness of walnuts and the herbaceousness of basil.
Preparation Time: 10 minutes
Total Time: 10 minutes
Serving: 1 cup
Ingredients
1/2 cup walnuts
1 cup fresh basil leaves
1 garlic clove
Juice of 1 lemon
2 tablespoons nutritional yeast
1/4 cup olive oil
Water, as needed
Instructions
1. In a food processor, combine walnuts, basil leaves, garlic clove, lemon juice, nutritional yeast, and olive oil.
2. Pulse until well combined and a thick paste forms.
3. Thin the dressing with water to reach desired consistency.

4. Serve immediately over salads or store in an airtight container in the refrigerator for up to one week.
Nutritional Info: Calories: 140, Protein: 4g, Carbohydrates: 3g, Fat: 14g, Fiber: 1g

Chickpea Tahini Dressing

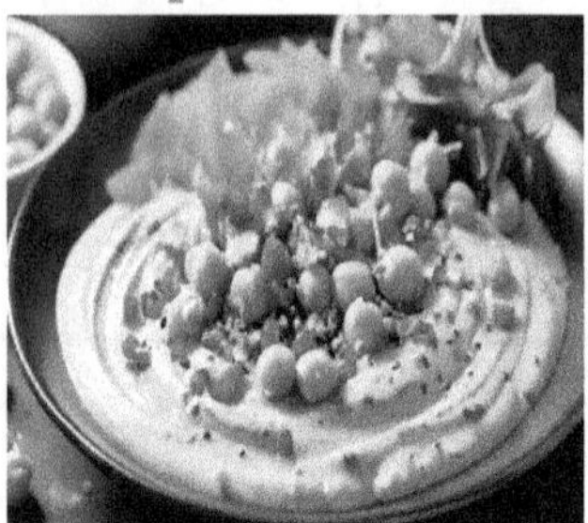

A creamy and protein-packed dressing with the nuttiness of tahini and the earthiness of chickpeas.
Preparation Time: 5 minutes
Total Time: 5 minutes
Serving: 1/2 cup
Ingredients
1/4 cup tahini
1/4 cup cooked chickpeas
Juice of 1 lemon
1 garlic clove, minced
Water, as needed
Instruction
1. In a blender, combine tahini, cooked chickpeas, lemon juice, and minced garlic.
2. Blend until smooth, adding water as needed to reach desired consistency.
3. Serve immediately over salads or store in an airtight container in the refrigerator for up to one week.
Nutritional Info: Calories: 120, Protein: 5g, Carbohydrates: 6g, Fat: 9g, Fiber: 2g

Avocado Cilantro Lime

A creamy and zesty dressing with the richness of avocado and the freshness of cilantro and lime.
Preparation Time: 5 minutes
Total Time: 5 minutes
Serving: 3/4 cup
Ingredients
1 ripe avocado
Juice of 2 limes
1/4 cup fresh cilantro leaves
1 garlic clove, minced
Water, as needed
Instructions
1. In a blender, combine ripe avocado, lime juice, cilantro leaves, and minced garlic.
2. Blend until smooth, adding water as needed to reach desired consistency.

3. Serve immediately over salads or store in an airtight container in the refrigerator for up to one week.
Nutritional Info: Calories: 90, Protein: 2g, Carbohydrates: 7g, Fat: 7g, Fiber: 3g

Sesame Ginger Miso Dressing

A bold and flavorful dressing with the nuttiness of sesame, the umami of miso, and the zing of ginger.

Preparation Time: 10 minutes
Total Time: 10 minutes
Serving: 1/2 cup

Ingredients

2 tablespoons tahini
1 tablespoon white miso paste
1 tablespoon rice vinegar
1 teaspoon grated fresh ginger
1 garlic clove, minced
1 tablespoon tamari or soy sauce
Water, as needed

Instructions

1. In a small bowl, whisk together tahini, white miso paste, rice vinegar, grated fresh ginger, minced garlic, and tamari or soy sauce.
2. Thin the dressing with water to reach desired consistency.
3. Serve immediately over salads or store in an airtight container in the refrigerator for up to one week.
Nutritional Info: Calories: 80, Protein: 3g, Carbohydrates: 5g, Fat: 6g, Fiber: 1g

Sunflower Seed Ranch

A creamy and herby dressing with the richness of sunflower seeds and classic ranch flavors.

Preparation Time: 10 minutes
Total Time: 10 minutes
Serving: 1 cup

Ingredients

1/2 cup raw sunflower seeds, soaked for at least 2 hours
1/4 cup water
Juice of 1 lemon
2 tablespoons chopped fresh dill
2 tablespoons chopped fresh chives
1 garlic clove, minced

Instructions

1. In a blender, combine soaked sunflower seeds, water, lemon juice, chopped fresh dill, chopped fresh chives, and minced garlic.
2. Blend until smooth and creamy.
3. Serve immediately over salads or store in an airtight container in the refrigerator for up to one week.
Nutritional Info: Calories: 120, Protein: 5g, Carbohydrates: 5g, Fat: 9g, Fiber: 2g

Pumpkin Seed Cilantro Lime

A vibrant and flavorful dressing with the nuttiness of pumpkin seeds and the freshness of cilantro and lime.

Preparation Time: 5 minutes

Total Time: 5 minutes

Serving: 1/2 cup

Ingredients

1/4 cup pumpkin seeds (pepitas)

Juice of 1 lime

1/4 cup fresh cilantro leaves

1 garlic clove, minced

2 tablespoons olive oil

Water, as needed

Instructions

1. In a blender, combine pumpkin seeds, lime juice, cilantro leaves, minced garlic, and olive oil.

2. Blend until smooth, adding water as needed to reach desired consistency.

3. Serve immediately over salads or store in an airtight container in the refrigerator for up to one week.

Nutritional Info: Calories: 100, Protein: 4g, Carbohydrates: 3g, Fat: 8g, Fiber: 1g

Roasted Red Pepper Walnut

A smoky and nutty dressing with the sweetness of roasted red peppers and the richness of walnuts.

Preparation Time: 15 minutes

Total Time: 15 minutes

Serving: 1 cup

Ingredients

1/2 cup walnuts

1 roasted red pepper, peeled and seeded

1 garlic clove

Juice of 1 lemon

2 tablespoons olive oil

Water, as needed

Instructions

1. In a food processor, combine walnuts, roasted red pepper, garlic clove, lemon juice, and olive oil.

2. Pulse until smooth, adding water as needed to reach desired consistency.

3. Serve immediately over salads or store in an airtight container in the refrigerator for up to one week.

Nutritional Info: Calories: 140, Protein: 3g, Carbohydrates: 5g, Fat: 12g, Fiber: 2g

Peanut Lime Dressing

A tangy and nutty dressing with the richness of peanuts and the brightness of lime.

Preparation Time: 5 minutes

Total Time: 5 minutes

Serving: 1/2 cup
Ingredients
1/4 cup peanut butter
Juice of 1 lime
1 tablespoon tamari or soy sauce
1 tablespoon maple syrup or agave syrup
1 garlic clove, minced
Water, as needed
Instructions
1. In a small bowl, whisk together peanut butter, lime juice, tamari or soy sauce,
maple syrup or agave syrup, and minced garlic.
2. Thin the dressing with water to reach desired consistency.
3. Serve immediately over salads or store in an airtight container in the refrigerator
for up to one week.
Nutritional Info: Calories: 120, Protein: 5g, Carbohydrates: 7g, Fat: 9g, Fiber: 2g

Sesame Orange Dressing

A citrusy and nutty dressing with the sweetness of orange and the nuttiness of sesame.
Preparation Time: 5 minutes
Total Time: 5 minutes
Serving: Makes about 1/2 cup
Ingredients:
2 tablespoons tahini
Juice of 1 orange
1 tablespoon rice vinegar
1 tablespoon tamari or soy sauce
1 teaspoon maple syrup or agave syrup
1 teaspoon grated fresh ginger
Water, as needed
Instructions
1. In a small bowl, whisk together tahini, orange juice, rice vinegar, tamari or soy
sauce, maple syrup or agave syrup, and grated fresh ginger.
2. Thin the dressing with water to reach desired consistency.
3. Serve immediately over salads or store in an airtight container in the refrigerator
for up to one week.
Nutritional Info: Calories: 100, Protein: 3g, Carbohydrates: 6g, Fat: 8g, Fiber: 2g

White Bean Rosemary

A creamy and herby dressing with the creaminess of white beans and the aroma of rosemary.
Preparation Time: 10 minutes
Total Time: 10 minutes
Serving: 1 cup
Ingredients
1/2 cup cooked white beans
1 tablespoon fresh rosemary leaves
Juice of 1 lemon

1 garlic clove, minced
2 tablespoons olive oil
Water, as needed
Instructions
1. In a blender, combine cooked white beans, rosemary leaves, lemon juice, minced garlic, and olive oil.
2. Blend until smooth, adding water as needed to reach desired consistency.
3. Serve immediately over salads or store in an airtight container in the refrigerator for up to one week.
Nutritional Info: Calories: 110, Protein: 4g, Carbohydrates: 7g, Fat: 7g, Fiber: 2g
Mango Lime Dressing

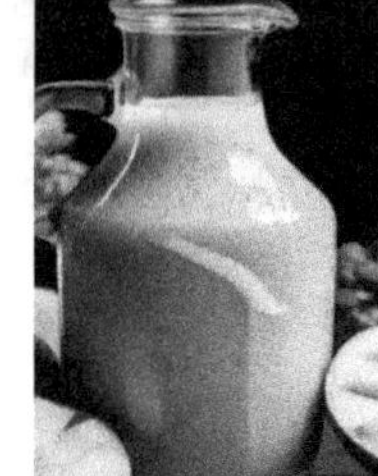

A tropical and tangy dressing with the sweetness of mango and the brightness of lime.
Preparation Time: 5 minutes
Total Time: 5 minutes
Serving: 3/4 cup
Ingredients
1 ripe mango, peeled and diced
Juice of 2 limes
1 tablespoon olive oil
1 tablespoon maple syrup or agave syrup
Pinch of chili flakes (optional)
Water, as needed
Instructions
1. In a blender, combine diced mango, lime juice, olive oil, maple syrup or agave syrup, and chili flakes (if using).
2. Blend until smooth, adding water as needed to reach desired consistency.
3. Serve immediately over salads or store in an airtight container in the refrigerator for up to one week.
Nutritional Info: Calories: 90, Protein: 1g, Carbohydrates: 15g, Fat: 4g, Fiber: 2g

Black Bean Chipotle Dressing

A smoky and spicy dressing with the creaminess of black beans and the heat of chipotle peppers.
Preparation Time: 10 minutes
Total Time: 10 minutes
Serving: 1 cup
Ingredients
1/2 cup cooked black beans
1 chipotle pepper in adobo sauce

Juice of 1 lime
1 garlic clove
2 tablespoons olive oil
Water, as needed
Instructions
1. In a blender, combine cooked black beans, chipotle pepper in adobo sauce, lime juice, garlic clove, and olive oil.
2. Blend until smooth, adding water as needed to reach desired consistency.
3. Serve immediately over salads or store in an airtight container in the refrigerator for up to one week.
Nutritional Info: Calories: 120, Protein: 4g, Carbohydrates: 9g, Fat: 8g, Fiber: 3g

Balsamic Vinaigrette

A classic dressing with tangy balsamic vinegar and savory herbs.
Preparation Time: 5 minutes
Total Time: 5 minutes
Serving: 1 cup
Ingredients
1/2 cup extra virgin olive oil
1/4 cup balsamic vinegar
1 tablespoon Dijon mustard
1 garlic clove, minced
Salt and pepper to taste
Instructions
1. In a small bowl, whisk together oil, balsamic vinegar, minced garlic, Dijon mustard, salt, and pepper until well combined.
2. Adjust seasoning according to taste preference.
3. Serve immediately over salads or store in an airtight container in the refrigerator for up to one week.
Nutritional Info: Calories: 120, Protein: 0g, Carbohydrates: 3g, Fat: 14g, Fiber: 0g

Creamy Avocado Cilantro Dressing

A creamy and flavorful dressing featuring avocado and fresh cilantro.
Preparation Time: 5 minutes
Total Time: 5 minutes
Serving: 1 cup
Ingredients
1 ripe avocado, peeled and pitted
1/4 cup fresh cilantro leaves
Juice of 1 lime
1/4 cup water
1 tablespoon olive oil
1 garlic clove, minced
Salt and pepper to taste
Instructions

1. In a blender or food processor, combine ripe avocado, cilantro leaves, lime juice, water, olive oil, minced garlic, salt, and pepper.
2. Blend until smooth and creamy.
3. Adjust seasoning according to taste preference.
4. Serve immediately over salads or store in an airtight container in the refrigerator for up to three days.
Nutritional Info: Calories: 80, Protein: 1g, Carbohydrates: 5g, Fat: 7g, Fiber: 3g

Maple Dijon Dressing

A sweet and tangy dressing with the perfect balance of maple syrup and Dijon mustard.
Preparation Time: 5 minutes
Total Time: 5 minutes
Serving: 1/2 cup
Ingredients
3 tablespoons extra virgin olive oil
2 tablespoons apple cider vinegar
1 tablespoon Dijon mustard
1 tablespoon maple syrup
1 garlic clove, minced
Salt and pepper to taste
Instructions
1. In a small bowl, whisk together olive oil, apple cider vinegar, Dijon mustard, maple syrup, minced garlic, salt, and pepper until well combined.
2. Adjust seasoning according to taste preference.
3. Serve immediately over salads or store in an airtight container in the refrigerator for up to one week.
Nutritional Info: Calories: 120, Protein: 0g, Carbohydrates: 5g, Fat: 12g, Fiber: 0g

Ginger Sesame Dressing

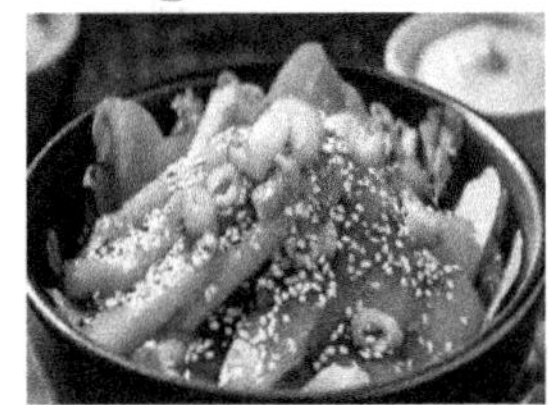

A zesty and aromatic dressing with the flavors of fresh ginger and toasted sesame oil.
Preparation Time: 5 minutes
Total Time: 5 minutes
Serving: 3/4 cup
Ingredients
1/4 cup rice vinegar
2 tablespoons tamari or soy sauce
1 tablespoon maple syrup or agave syrup
1 tablespoon toasted sesame oil
1 tablespoon grated fresh ginger

1 garlic clove, minced
2 tablespoons water
Instructions
1. In a small bowl, whisk together rice vinegar, tamari or soy sauce, maple syrup or agave syrup, toasted sesame oil, grated fresh ginger, minced garlic, and water until well combined.
2. Adjust seasoning according to taste preference.
3. Serve immediately over salads or store in an airtight container in the refrigerator for up to one week.
Nutritional Info: Calories: 60, Protein: 1g, Carbohydrates: 7g, Fat: 3g, Fiber: 0g

Lemon Herb Dressing

A bright and herby dressing with fresh lemon juice and aromatic herbs.
Preparation Time: 5 minutes
Total Time: 5 minutes
Serving: 1/2 cup
Ingredients
1/4 cup extra virgin olive oil
Juice of 1 lemon
2 tablespoons chopped fresh herbs (such as parsley, basil, or dill)
1 garlic clove, minced
Salt and pepper to taste
Instructions
1. In a small bowl, whisk together olive oil, lemon juice, chopped fresh herbs, minced garlic, salt, and pepper until well combined.
2. Adjust seasoning according to taste preference.
3. Serve immediately over salads or store in an airtight container in the refrigerator for up to one week.
Nutritional Info: Calories: 120, Protein: 0g, Carbohydrates: 2g, Fat: 14g, Fiber: 0g

Cilantro Lime Dressing

A zesty and vibrant dressing with the flavors of fresh cilantro and lime.
Preparation Time: 5 minutes
Total Time: 5 minutes
Serving: 1/2 cup
Ingredients
1/4 cup extra virgin olive oil
Juice of 2 limes
2 tablespoons chopped fresh cilantro
1 garlic clove, minced
Salt and pepper to taste
Instructions
1. In a small bowl, whisk together olive oil, lime juice, chopped fresh cilantro, minced garlic, salt, and pepper until well combined.
2. Adjust seasoning according to taste preference.

3. Serve immediately over salads or store in an airtight container in the refrigerator for up to one week.
Nutritional Info: Calories: 120, Protein: 0g, Carbohydrates: 2g, Fat: 14g, Fiber: 0g

Tahini Miso Dressing

A creamy and umami-rich dressing made with tahini and miso paste.
Preparation Time: 5 minutes
Total Time: 5 minutes
Serving: 1/2 cup
Ingredients
1/4 cup tahini
2 tablespoons white miso paste
2 tablespoons rice vinegar
1 tablespoon maple syrup or agave syrup
1 garlic clove, minced
2 tablespoons water
Instructions
1. In a small bowl, whisk together tahini, white miso paste, rice vinegar, maple syrup or agave syrup, minced garlic, and water until smooth and creamy.
2. Adjust consistency by adding more water if desired.
3. Serve immediately over salads or store in an airtight container in the refrigerator for up to one week.
Nutritional Info: Calories: 80, Protein: 2g, Carbohydrates: 6g, Fat: 6g, Fiber: 1g

Sun-Dried Tomato Basil Dressing

A tangy and aromatic dressing with the sweetness of sun-dried tomatoes and the freshness of basil.
Preparation Time: 10 minutes
Total Time: 10 minutes
Serving: 3/4 cup
Ingredients
1/4 cup sun-dried tomatoes (packed in oil), drained
1/4 cup packed fresh basil leaves
2 tablespoons red wine vinegar
1 garlic clove, minced
1/4 cup extra virgin olive oil
Salt and pepper to taste
Instructions
1. In a blender or food processor, combine sun-dried tomatoes, fresh basil leaves, red wine vinegar, minced garlic, and olive oil.
2. Blend until smooth.
3. Season with salt and pepper to taste.
4. Serve immediately over salads or store in an airtight container in the refrigerator for up to one week.
Nutritional Info: Calories: 140, Protein: 1g, Carbohydrates: 5g, Fat: 14g, Fiber: 1g

Honey Mustard Dressing

A sweet and tangy dressing with the perfect balance of honey and mustard flavors.
Preparation Time: 5 minutes
Total Time: 5 minutes
Serving: 1/2 cup
Ingredients
1/4 cup extra virgin olive oil
2 tablespoons apple cider vinegar
1 tablespoon Dijon mustard
1 tablespoon honey or agave syrup
1 garlic clove, minced
Salt and pepper to taste
Instructions
1. In a small bowl, whisk together olive oil, apple cider vinegar, Dijon mustard, honey or agave syrup, minced garlic, salt, and pepper until well combined.
2. Adjust seasoning according to taste preference.
3. Serve immediately over salads or store in an airtight container in the refrigerator for up to one week.
Nutritional Info: Calories: 120, Protein: 0g, Carbohydrates: 6g, Fat: 14g, Fiber: 0g

Greek Yogurt Ranch Dressing

A creamy and tangy dressing made with Greek yogurt and classic ranch herbs and spices.
Preparation Time: 5 minutes
Total Time: 5 minutes
Serving: 1 cup
Ingredients
1/2 cup plain Greek yogurt
2 tablespoons chopped fresh dill
2 tablespoons chopped fresh chives
1 garlic clove, minced
1 tablespoon apple cider vinegar
1 tablespoon olive oil
Salt and pepper to taste
Instructions
1. In a small bowl, whisk together Greek yogurt, chopped fresh dill, chopped fresh chives, minced garlic, apple cider vinegar, olive oil, salt, and pepper until well combined.
2. Adjust seasoning according to taste preference.
3. Serve immediately over salads or store in an airtight container in the refrigerator for up to one week.
Nutritional Info: Calories: 90, Protein: 4g, Carbohydrates: 3g, Fat: 7g, Fiber: 0g

Spicy Peanut Dressing

A bold and flavorful dressing with the nuttiness of peanut butter and a kick of spice.
Preparation Time: 5 minutes

Total Time: 5 minutes
Serving: 1/2 cup
Ingredients
1/4 cup peanut butter
2 tablespoons rice vinegar
1 tablespoon tamari or soy sauce
1 tablespoon maple syrup or agave syrup
1 teaspoon grated fresh ginger
1 garlic clove, minced
2 tablespoons water
Pinch of red pepper flakes (optional)
Instructions
1. In a small bowl, whisk together peanut butter, rice vinegar, tamari or soy sauce, maple syrup or agave syrup, grated fresh ginger, minced garlic, water, and red pepper flakes (if using) until smooth and creamy.
2. Adjust consistency by adding more water if desired.
3. Serve immediately over salads or store in an airtight container in the refrigerator for up to one week.
Nutritional Info: Calories: 130, Protein: 4g, Carbohydrates: 7g, Fat: 10g, Fiber: 1g

Creamy Lemon Poppy Seed Dressing

A creamy and citrusy dressing with the crunch of poppy seeds.
Preparation Time: 5 minutes
Total Time: 5 minutes
Serving: 1/2 cup
Ingredients
1/4 cup plain Greek yogurt
Juice of 1 lemon
1 tablespoon maple syrup or agave syrup
1 teaspoon poppy seeds
1 garlic clove, minced
Salt and pepper to taste
Instructions
1. In a small bowl, whisk together Greek yogurt, lemon juice, maple syrup or agave syrup, poppy seeds, minced garlic, salt, and pepper until well combined.
2. Adjust seasoning according to taste preference.
3. Serve immediately over salads or store in an airtight container in the refrigerator for up to one week.
Nutritional Info: Calories: 60, Protein: 3g, Carbohydrates: 7g, Fat: 3g, Fiber: 0g

DRINK

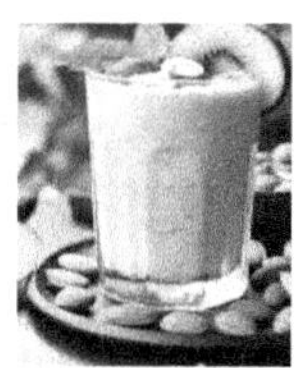

Almond Banana Smoothie

A creamy and satisfying smoothie with the goodness of almonds and bananas.
Preparation Time: 5 minutes
Total Time: 5 minutes
Servings: 2
Ingredients
2 ripe bananas
1 cup almond milk
1/4 cup almonds
1 tablespoon maple syrup
1/2 teaspoon vanilla extract
Instructions
1. In a blender, combine ripe bananas, almond milk, almonds, maple syrup, and vanilla extract.
2. Blend the mixture until smooth and creamy.
3. Divide the smoothie into glasses and serve right away.
Nutritional Info: Calories: 250, Protein: 5g, Carbohydrates: 40g, Fat: 8g, Fiber: 4g

Chia Seed Green Smoothie

A nutrient-packed green smoothie enriched with chia seeds for added fiber and omega-3s.
Preparation Time: 5 minutes
Total Time: 5 minutes
Servings: 2
Ingredients
2 cups spinach
1 ripe avocado
1 tablespoon chia seeds
1 cup coconut water
Juice of 1 lime
Instructions
1. In a blender bowl, combine spinach, chia seeds, ripe avocado, lime juice and coconut water. Blend until smooth
3. Divide smoothie among two serving glasses and serve immediately.
Nutritional Info: Calories: 220, Protein: 6g, Carbohydrates: 15g, Fat: 15g, Fiber: 10g

Carrot Ginger Turmeric Juice

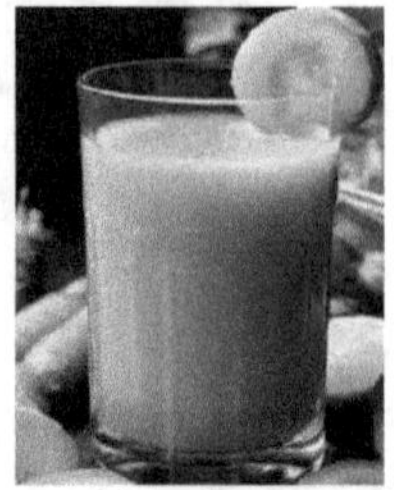

A vibrant juice bursting with the flavors and health benefits of carrots, ginger, and turmeric.
Preparation Time: 10 minutes
Total Time: 10 minutes
Servings: 2
Ingredients
4 large carrots, peeled and chopped
1-inch piece of fresh ginger, peeled
1 teaspoon ground turmeric
1 tablespoon lemon juice
2 cups water
Ice cubes (optional)
Instructions
1. In a juicer, juice the carrots and ginger.
2. Transfer the juice to a blender and add ground turmeric, lemon juice, and water.
3. Blend until smooth.
4. Serve over ice, if desired.
Nutritional Info: Calories: 90, Protein: 2g, Carbohydrates: 20g, Fat: 0g, Fiber: 6g

Quinoa Berry Smoothie

A protein-rich smoothie featuring quinoa and mixed berries for a delicious and filling drink.
Preparation Time: 10 minutes
Total Time: 10 minutes
Servings: 2
Ingredients
1/2 cup cooked quinoa, cooled
1 cup mixed berries (strawberries, blueberries, raspberries)
1 ripe banana
1 cup almond milk
1 tablespoon honey or agave syrup
Instructions
1. In a blender, combine cooked quinoa, mixed berries, ripe banana, almond milk, and honey or agave syrup.
2. Blend mixture until smooth.
3. Pour into two serving glasses and serve immediately.
Nutritional Info: Calories: 260, Protein: 6g, Carbohydrates: 50g, Fat: 4g, Fiber: 8g

Pumpkin Seed Milk

A creamy and nutty dairy-free milk made from pumpkin seeds, rich in nutrients like magnesium and zinc.

Preparation Time: 10 minutes

Total Time: 10 minutes

Servings: 4

Ingredients

1 cup raw pumpkin seeds (pepitas), soaked overnight

4 cups water

1 tablespoon agave syrup or maple syrup o (optional)

1 teaspoon vanilla extract (optional)

Instructions

1. Drain and rinse soaked pumpkin seeds.

2. In a blender, combine soaked pumpkin seeds and water.

3. Blend on high until smooth.

4. Strain the mixture through a nut milk bag or fine mesh sieve, squeezing out as much liquid as possible.

5. Add maple syrup or agave syrup and vanilla extract, if using.

6. Transfer pumpkin seed milk to a glass jar and refrigerate. Shake well before serving.

Nutritional Info: Calories: 150, Protein: 5g, Carbohydrates: 3g, Fat: 13g, Fiber: 1g

Cucumber Mint Gazpacho

A refreshing and cooling soup made with cucumber, mint, and other fresh ingredients.

Preparation Time: 15 minutes

Chilling Time: 1 hour

Total Time: 1 hour 15 minutes

Servings: 4

Ingredients

2 large cucumbers, peeled and chopped

1 green bell pepper, seeded and chopped

1/2 red onion, chopped

2 cloves garlic, minced

1/4 cup fresh mint leaves

2 tablespoons lemon juice

2 tablespoons olive oil

Salt and pepper, to taste

Optional garnishes: chopped cucumber, mint leaves, drizzle of olive oil

Instructions

1. In a blender, combine chopped cucumbers, green bell pepper, red onion, minced garlic, fresh mint leaves, lemon juice, and olive oil.

2. Blend until smooth.

3. Season with salt and pepper to taste.

4. Transfer the gazpacho to a large bowl and refrigerate for at least 1 hour to chill.

5. Before serving, stir the gazpacho and adjust seasoning if necessary.

6. Serve cold, garnished with chopped cucumber, mint leaves, and a drizzle of olive oil if desired.

Nutritional Info: Calories: 100, Protein: 2g, Carbohydrates: 10g, Fat: 7g, Fiber: 3g

Sesame Ginger Tofu Smoothie

A protein-packed smoothie featuring tofu, sesame seeds, and ginger for a unique and satisfying drink.

Preparation Time: 10 minutes
Total Time: 10 minutes
Servings: 2

Ingredients

1/2 block (about 7 ounces) firm tofu
2 tablespoons sesame seeds
1 tablespoon grated fresh ginger
1 ripe banana
1 cup almond milk
1 tablespoon honey or agave syrup

Instructions

1. In a blender, combine firm tofu, sesame seeds, grated fresh ginger, ripe banana, almond milk, and honey or agave syrup.
2. Blend until smooth and creamy.
3. Pour the smoothie into two glass cup and serve immediately.

Nutritional Info: Calories: 280, Protein: 14g, Carbohydrates: 30g, Fat: 14g, Fiber: 6g

Brown Rice Horchata

A creamy and refreshing rice-based drink flavored with cinnamon and vanilla.

Preparation Time: 10 minutes
Cooking Time: 20 minutes
Chilling Time: 2 hours
Total Time: 2 hours 30 minutes
Servings: 4

Ingredients

1 cup brown rice
4 cups water
1 cinnamon stick
1/4 cup maple syrup or agave syrup
1 teaspoon vanilla extract
Ground cinnamon, for garnish

Instructions

1. In a saucepan, combine brown rice, water, and cinnamon stick. Bring to a boil.
2. Reduce heat to low, cover, and simmer for 20 minutes, or until rice is tender.
3. Remove from heat and let it cool to room temperature.
4. Once cooled, discard the cinnamon stick and transfer the rice mixture to a blender.
5. Add maple syrup or agave syrup and vanilla extract.Blend until smooth.

6. Strain the mixture through a nut milk bag or fine mesh sieve, squeezing out as much liquid as possible.
7. Transfer the horchata to a pitcher and refrigerate for at least 2 hours to chill.
8. Before serving, stir the horchata and pour into glasses.
9. Sprinkle ground cinnamon on top for garnish.
Nutritional Info: Calories: 180, Protein: 3g, Carbohydrates: 35g, Fat: 2g, Fiber: 2g

Sunflower Seed Butter Smoothie

A creamy and nutty smoothie made with sunflower seed butter and bananas for a delicious and energizing drink.
Preparation Time: 5 minutes
Total Time: 5 minutes
Servings: 2
Ingredients
2 ripe bananas
2 tablespoons sunflower seed butter
1 cup almond milk
1 tablespoon maple syrup or agave syrup
1/2 teaspoon ground cinnamon
Instructions
1. In a blender, combine ripe bananas, sunflower seed butter, almond milk, maple syrup or agave syrup, and ground cinnamon.
2. Blend until smooth and creamy.
3. Pour the smoothie among two serving glass cup and serve immediately.
Nutritional Info: Calories: 280, Protein: 6g, Carbohydrates: 35g, Fat: 15g, Fiber: 6g

Hemp Seed Berry Smoothie

A protein-rich smoothie featuring hemp seeds and mixed berries for a nutritious and satisfying drink.
Preparation Time: 5 minutes
Total Time: 5 minutes
Servings: 2
Ingredients
1 cup mixed berries (strawberries, blueberries, raspberries)
1 ripe banana
2 tablespoons hemp seeds
1 cup coconut water
1 tablespoon honey or agave syrup
Instructions
1. In a blender, combine mixed berries, ripe banana, hemp seeds, coconut water, and honey or agave syrup.
2. Blend until smooth.
3. Pour the smoothie into glasses and serve immediately.
Nutritional Info: Calories: 230, Protein: 5g, Carbohydrates: 40g, Fat: 8g, Fiber: 8g

Oat Milk Latte

A creamy and dairy-free latte made with homemade oat milk for a comforting and delicious beverage.

Preparation Time: 10 minutes
Cooking Time: 5 minutes
Total Time: 15 minutes
Servings: 2

Ingredients

1/2 cup rolled oats
4 cups water
2 shots espresso or 1/2 cup strong brewed coffee
1 tablespoon maple syrup (optional)
Pinch of ground cinnamon (optional)

Instructions

1. In a blender, combine rolled oats and water.
2. Blend on high until smooth.
3. Strain the oat milk through a nut milk bag or fine mesh sieve, squeezing out as much liquid as possible.
4. Transfer oat milk to a small saucepan and heat over medium heat until warmed through.
5. Meanwhile, prepare espresso or strong brewed coffee.
6. Divide the oat milk between two mugs and add a shot of espresso or half of the brewed coffee to each mug.
7. Stir in maple syrup or agave syrup and ground cinnamon, if using.
8. Serve hot and enjoy.

Nutritional Info: Calories: 100, Protein: 3g, Carbohydrates: 20g, Fat: 2g, Fiber: 4g

Peanut Butter Banana Smoothie Bowl

A thick and creamy smoothie bowl made with peanut butter, bananas, and topped with crunchy granola and fresh fruit.

Preparation Time: 5 minutes
Total Time: 5 minutes
Servings: 2

Ingredients

2 ripe bananas
2 tablespoons peanut butter
1/2 cup almond milk
1 tablespoon honey or agave syrup
Toppings: granola, sliced banana, berries, shredded coconut

Instructions

1. In a blender, combine ripe bananas, peanut butter, almond milk, and honey or agave syrup.
2. Blend until smooth and creamy.
3. Pour the smoothie into bowls.
4. Top with granola, sliced banana, berries, and shredded coconut.
5. Serve immediately and enjoy with a spoon.

Nutritional Info: Calories: 300, Protein: 7g, Carbohydrates: 40g, Fat: 14g, Fiber: 6g

Green Goddess Smoothie

A refreshing and nutrient-packed smoothie bursting with green goodness.
Preparation Time: 5 minutes
Total Time: 5 minutes
Servings: 2
Ingredients
2 cups spinach
1 ripe banana
1 cup almond milk
1 tablespoon chia seeds
1 tablespoon almond butter
1/2 cup frozen pineapple chunks
Instructions
1. Combine all ingredients in a blender.
2. Blend until smooth.
3. Divide smoothie among two serving glass cups and serve immediately.
Nutritional Info: Calories: 180, Protein: 5g, Carbohydrates: 25g, Fat: 8g, Fiber: 6g

Berry Blast Smoothie

A vibrant and antioxidant-rich smoothie featuring a medley of berries.
Preparation Time: 5 minutes
Total Time: 5 minutes
Servings: 2
Ingredients
1 cup mixed berries (strawberries, blueberries, raspberries)
1 ripe banana
1 cup coconut water
1 tablespoon flaxseeds
1/2 cup spinach
Instructions
1. Place all ingredients in a blender.
2. Blend until smooth.
3. Pour the smoothie into two glass cups and serve immediately.
Nutritional Info: Calories: 150, Protein: 4g, Carbohydrates: 30g, Fat: 3g, Fiber: 8g

Golden Turmeric Latte

A warming and anti-inflammatory drink infused with the goodness of turmeric.
Preparation Time: 5 minutes
Cooking Time: 5 minutes
Total Time: 10 minutes
Servings: 2
Ingredients
2 cups almond milk

1 teaspoon ground turmeric
1/2 teaspoon ground cinnamon
1/4 teaspoon ground ginger
1 tablespoon maple syrup
Pinch of black pepper

Instructions

1. Heat the almond milk in a saucepan over medium-high heat.
2. Whisk in turmeric, cinnamon, ginger, maple syrup, and black pepper.
3. Continue to heat for 5 minutes, stirring occasionally.
4. Pour into mugs and serve hot.

Nutritional Info: Calories: 100, Protein: 2g, Carbohydrates: 15g, Fat: 4g, Fiber: 1g

Creamy Avocado Smoothie

A creamy and satisfying smoothie enriched with avocado's healthy fats.

Preparation Time: 5 minutes
Total Time: 5 minutes
Servings: 2

Ingredients

1 ripe avocado
1 cup spinach
1 cup coconut water
1 tablespoon honey or agave syrup
Juice of 1 lime
1/2 cup frozen mango chunks

Instructions

1. Scoop out the flesh of the avocado and add it to a blender.
2. Add spinach, coconut water, honey or agave syrup, lime juice, and frozen mango.
3. Blend until smooth.
4. Pour the smoothie into two serving glasses and serve immediately.

Nutritional Info: Calories: 220, Protein: 3g, Carbohydrates: 30g, Fat: 10g, Fiber: 8g

Chocolate Peanut Butter Protein Shake

A decadent and protein-packed shake for a post-workout boost.

Preparation Time: 5 minutes
Total Time: 5 minutes
Serving: 1

Ingredients

1 cup almond milk
1 scoop chocolate protein powder (plant-based)
1 tablespoon peanut butter
1 tablespoon cocoa powder
1/2 frozen banana
Ice cubes (optional)

Instructions

1. In a blender, combine almond milk, protein powder, peanut butter, cocoa powder, frozen banana, and ice cubes if using.

2. Blend until smooth and creamy.

3. Transfer to a serving glass cup and enjoy immediately.

Nutritional Info: Calories: 300, Protein: 25g, Carbohydrates: 20g, Fat: 12g, Fiber: 6g

Matcha Green Tea Latte

A frothy and energizing drink infused with the goodness of matcha.

Preparation Time: 5 minutes

Cooking Time: 5 minutes

Total Time: 10 minutes

Serving: 1

Ingredients

1 teaspoon matcha powder

1 cup almond milk

1 tablespoon maple syrup

Instructions

1. In a small saucepan, heat almond milk over medium heat until steaming.

2. In a mug, whisk together matcha powder and maple syrup.

3. Pour the hot almond milk over the matcha mixture.

4. Use a frother to blend until frothy.

5. Serve hot and enjoy.

Nutritional Info: Calories: 100, Protein: 3g, Carbohydrates: 20g, Fat: 3g, Fiber: 1g

Pineapple Coconut Smoothie

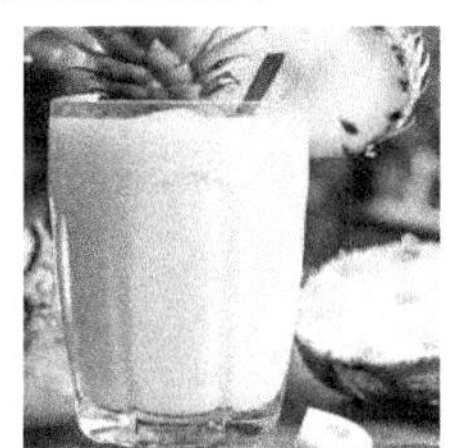

A tropical delight featuring the flavors of pineapple and coconut.

Preparation Time: 5 minutes

Total Time: 5 minutes

Servings: 2

Ingredients

1 cup frozen pineapple chunks

1 ripe banana

1/2 cup coconut milk

1/2 cup coconut water

1 tablespoon shredded coconut

1 tablespoon lime juice

Instructions

1. Combine all ingredients in a blender.

2. Blend until smooth.

3. Pour the smoothie into 2 serving glass cups and serve immediately.

Nutritional Info: Calories: 180, Protein: 2g, Carbohydrates: 30g, Fat: 8g, Fiber: 4g

Spicy Ginger Lemonade

A zesty and refreshing lemonade with a kick of spicy ginger.
Preparation Time: 10 minutes
Total Time: 10 minutes
Servings: 2
Ingredients
2 cups cold water
Juice of 4 lemons
2 tablespoons maple syrup
1 tablespoon grated ginger
Pinch of cayenne pepper
Instructions
1. In a pitcher, combine cold water, lemon juice, maple syrup, grated ginger, and cayenne pepper.
2. Stir well to combine.
3. Serve over ice and garnish with lemon slices, if desired.
Nutritional Info: Calories: 80, Protein: 1g, Carbohydrates: 20g, Fat: 0g, Fiber: 1g

Vanilla Almond Milkshake

A classic milkshake with a dairy-free twist, flavored with vanilla and almond.
Preparation Time: 5 minutes
Total Time: 5 minutes
Servings: 2
Ingredients
2 cups almond milk
1 teaspoon vanilla extract
2 tablespoons maple syrup
1/2 cup ice cubes
Instructions
1. In a blender, combine almond milk, vanilla extract, maple syrup, and ice cubes.
2. Blend until smooth and frothy.
3. Divide among two serving glasses and serve immediately.
Nutritional Info: Calories: 100, Protein: 1g, Carbohydrates: 15g, Fat: 4g, Fiber: 0g

Raspberry Chia Seed Lemonade

A refreshing lemonade with the added health benefits of chia seeds and raspberries.
Preparation Time: 10 minutes
Total Time: 10 minutes
Servings: 2
Ingredients
2 cups cold water
Juice of 2 lemons
2 tablespoons maple syrup
2 tablespoons chia seeds
1/2 cup fresh raspberries

Instructions

1. In a pitcher, combine cold water, lemon juice, maple syrup, and chia seeds.
2. Stir the mixture well to combine and let it sit for 5 minutes.
3. Add fresh raspberries and stir again.
4. Serve over ice and enjoy.

Nutritional Info: Calories: 100, Protein: 2g, Carbohydrates: 20g, Fat: 3g, Fiber: 6g

Coconut Mango Lassi

A tropical twist on the traditional Indian yogurt-based drink.

Preparation Time: 5 minutes

Total Time: 5 minutes

Servings: 2

Ingredients

1 ripe mango, peeled and diced

1 cup coconut yogurt

1/2 cup coconut milk

1 tablespoon maple syrup

Pinch of cardamom powder

Instructions

1. In a blender, combine diced mango, coconut yogurt, coconut milk, maple syrup, and cardamom powder.
2. Blend until smooth and creamy.
3. Pour into glasses and serve chilled.

Nutritional Info: Calories: 200, Protein: 3g, Carbohydrates: 30g, Fat: 8g, Fiber: 4g

Cucumber Mint Cooler

A refreshing and hydrating drink with the cooling flavors of cucumber and mint.

Preparation Time: 10 minutes

Total Time: 10 minutes

Servings: 2

Ingredients

1 cucumber, peeled and chopped

Handful of fresh mint leaves

Juice of 1 lime

2 cups cold water

2 tablespoons agave syrup or honey

Ice cubes

Instructions

1. In a blender, combine chopped cucumber, mint leaves, lime juice, cold water, and agave syrup or honey.
2. Blend until smooth.
3. Strain to remove any pulp with a fine mesh sieve.
4. Garnish with mint leaves, serve over ice and enjoy!.

Nutritional Info: Calories: 60, Protein: 1g, Carbohydrates: 15g, Fat: 0g, Fiber: 2g

Peach Ginger Smoothie

A delightful blend of sweet peaches and spicy ginger for a refreshing beverage.
Preparation Time: 5 minutes
Total Time: 5 minutes
Servings: 2
Ingredients
2 ripe peaches, pitted and sliced
1 tablespoon grated ginger
1 cup almond milk
1 tablespoon honey or agave syrup
1/2 cup ice cubes
Instructions
1. In a blender, combine sliced peaches, grated ginger, almond milk, honey or agave syrup, and ice cubes.
2. Blend until smooth and creamy.
3. Divide smoothie among two serving glasses and enjoy immediately.
Nutritional Info: Calories: 120, Protein: 2g, Carbohydrates: 25g, Fat: 3g, Fiber: 4g

Tropical Green Smoothie

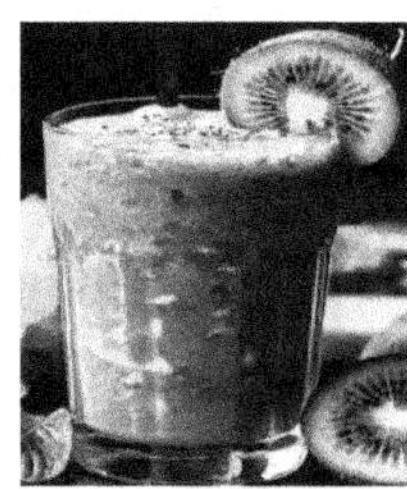

A tropical twist on the classic green smoothie, packed with vitamins and minerals.
Preparation Time: 5 minutes
Total Time: 5 minutes
Servings: 2
Ingredients
1 cup spinach
1/2 cup frozen pineapple chunks
1/2 cup frozen mango chunks
1 ripe banana
1 cup coconut water
1 tablespoon chia seeds
Instructions
1. Combine all ingredients in a blender.
2. Blend until smooth.
3. Pour into glasses and serve immediately.
Nutritional Info: Calories: 180, Protein: 4g, Carbohydrates: 35g, Fat: 4g, Fiber: 8g

Blueberry Oatmeal Smoothie

A hearty and filling smoothie featuring the goodness of oats and blueberries.
Preparation Time: 5 minutes
Total Time: 5 minutes
Servings: 2
Ingredients
1/2 cup rolled oats
1 cup almond milk
1 ripe banana
1 cup frozen blueberries
1 tablespoon almond butter
1 tablespoon maple syrup
Instructions
1. In a blender, combine rolled oats, almond milk, banana, frozen blueberries, almond butter, and maple syrup.
2. Blend until smooth and creamy.
3. Pour the smoothies into two serving glass cups and serve immediately.
Nutritional Info: Calories: 250, Protein: 6g, Carbohydrates: 45g, Fat: 6g, Fiber: 8g